PRAISE FOR M⸻

"Mackenzie does a beautiful ⸻
the perfect run and how we c⸻
basis. If you are looking for co⸻ ly
recommend⸻
Bestselling author and US Olympian, Ryan Hall

"Go ahead and chase perfection in your running, but understand that perfect is an experience, not an outcome. This is the message I took away from *The Perfect Run*, and I hope I never forget it."
Matt Fitzgerald, author of *Life Is a Marathon*

"Reading *The Perfect Run* is sure to increase your appreciation and enjoyment on the run, and that's a big payback."
Amby Burfoot, *Runner's World Magazine*

"In this age of distraction, we would all benefit from being more present more often. Mackenzie L. Havey shows how and why to achieve this goal in your running, and how that practice can benefit you in your non-running hours."
Scott Douglas, *Runner's World Magazine*

"Mindful running has changed my life for the better – when I'm feeling overwhelmed, stressed or anxious, pulling on my trainers is my form of therapy."
Huffington Post

"*Mindful Running* is the bridge to using your body, mind and surroundings to get the most out of your running…"
Deena Kastor, Olympic medallist and US marathon and half-marathon record holder

"From the very first page I was hooked. I loved this book."
Terry Pearson, leading mindfulness instructor

"A great read for anyone who, like us, struggles to fit running in around work and life, by explaining the benefits of taking the time out and running more mindfully, which has a great, positive impact on all areas of your life."
Run Deep Magazine

MACKENZIE L. HAVEY

THE
PERFECT
RUN

A Guide to Cultivating a
Near-Effortless Running State

BLOOMSBURY SPORT
LONDON · OXFORD · NEW YORK · NEW DELHI · SYDNEY

BLOOMSBURY SPORT
Bloomsbury Publishing Plc
50 Bedford Square, London, WC1B 3DP, UK

BLOOMSBURY, BLOOMSBURY SPORT and the Diana logo are trademarks of
Bloomsbury Publishing Plc

First published in Great Britain 2020

A catalogue record for this book is available from the British Library

Library of Congress Cataloguing-in-Publication data has been applied for

ISBN: PB: 978-1-4729-6865-4; eBook: 978-1-4729-6867-8; ePDF: 978-1-4729-6866-1

2 4 6 8 10 9 7 5 3 1

Typeset in ITC Giovanni Book by Deanta Global Publishing Services, Chennai, India
Printed and bound in Great Britain by CPI Group (UK) Ltd, Croydon CR0 4YY

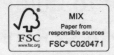

To find out more about our authors and books visit www.bloomsbury.com
and sign up for our newsletters

For Jason, Welly, Liesl, and Liv,
Always there to remind me
when to take my feet outside.

CONTENTS

INTRODUCTION

THE SHRILL BUGLE call of an elk horn sounds and 800 runners spring from the starting line. Aside from a delicate haze on the horizon and the vague smell of bonfire, there is little evidence of the countless wildfires burning across the western United States. Cowbells clang on either side of the trail lined with spectators clad in colorful insulated jackets, fitted trucker caps, and trail running shoes. I sport spandex capris and a paper-thin orange singlet with sunglasses and a hat that shades my face. The morning air fills my lungs and feels cool and crisp on my skin as we ascend our first climb.

It is Labor Day weekend 2017 and I am running the 6.8-mile (11-km) race that is part of The Rut mountain running series in Big Sky, Montana. The premier event, the 50K race, was the first U.S. race to be part of the International Skyrunning Series, bringing in some of the best of the best in ultra mountain running talent from around the world each year. Despite the shorter distance, the 11K race also attracts a crowd of supremely fit, hard-core athletes. Starting at Big Sky Resort's base area at around 7,500 feet (2,286 meters), it includes 1,700 feet (518 meters) of elevation gain and 1,700 feet (518 meters) of loss over single-track trails and rocky dirt roads.

Being a through-and-through flatlander from Minneapolis, this is a lung-busting amount of climbing for me, especially at altitude. Adding to the challenge is the fact that this is my initial race back after giving birth to my daughter, our firstborn. Her first birthday is just a few days away. While I ran through 40 weeks of pregnancy and had been back logging miles for months, I haven't stepped up to a race start line since Ironman Wisconsin almost two years prior. I feel out of my element both racing and being away from my daughter. While she is too young to understand it now, I remind myself that in a few years, seeing her mom run up mountains could make an impression.

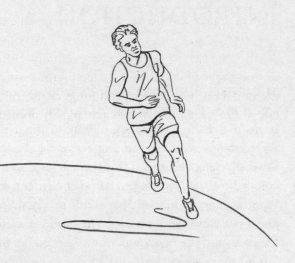

The "perfect" run can come in many shapes and forms.

As we scale the backside of Andesite Mountain on ski resort territory, the trail takes us over long climbing switchbacks. The biggest climb of the race starts in a tall grass alpine meadow around the first mile marker and doesn't top out until mile 5 (8 km), totaling 1,500 feet (457 meters) on that section. As we clamber upward, the line of runners slows for a moment, halted by the arresting beauty of the sun-soaked valley below. I think about how I want to bring my daughter to this spot one day.

With rocks and boulders on either side of the narrow trail of exposed ridgelines, I choose to follow the line of runners making their way up the mountain, occasionally passing or being passed. Around mile 4 (6.5 km), the switchback gets steeper and rockier before we move through a whitebark pine forest over bare loam that springs with each step. Hundreds of cutaneous receptors in my feet fire off sensory feedback in response to the changing terrain.

The light flickering through the trees on either side of the path has a focusing effect, heightening my awareness of every root and rock. The landscape is saturated with changing light, like an Impressionist painting. An elemental consciousness awakens within me as I glide through the passing moment.

Following a wider dirt road to the summit of Andesite Mountain, the location of the only aid station on the course, I feel a familiar exertional burn in my legs and lungs as the altitude deprives my body of oxygen. I forgot how remarkably nourishing this kind of hurt can feel. I gaze off into the distance as the dark outline of the 11,000-foot (3,353-meters) Lone Peak snaps into focus.

After hastily downing a cup of water, I let my legs take me down a dirt road to an abrupt turnoff that leads back into the outstretched branches of the forest. To descend on to the trail, I line up behind a few other runners and one by one we take hold of a thick, natural-fiber manila rope tied around a massive, ancient driftwood stump. I quickly lower myself down the steep embankment backward, feeling my hands burn over the stiff bristle as I reach the bottom and turn to run.

A sense of euphoria and propulsive energy takes hold. Cruising down the resort's lower ski runs, the air temperature rises. I pass a friendly, loquacious brook littered with dry logs and mountain detritus. Trees whisper by on either side and I precisely negotiate rocks and sudden turns almost without thinking. In this moment, my body and mind work in perfect tandem. It's as if I am under a hypnotic spell dictated by the rhythm of my feet and the sound of my breath.

Emerging from the trees, I scramble down the final descent over burrowed-out dirt footholds in the single track. I reenter a portal that leads back into my previous plane of existence, spitting me out within earshot of the brassy clangor of cowbells and blare of metal music. I feel like I am gliding without effort, maybe even flying, as I cross the finish line. In my happy exhaustion, I take stock of what has just unfolded. This, I know, is the perfect running experience.

* * *

The Paradox of Perfection

In the modern-day definition of the word, "perfection" generally denotes flawlessness. It's a condition in which a level of excellence can't be exceeded. A perfect test score is characterized by all correct answers to the questions on an exam. A perfect game in baseball is one during which a pitcher pitches at least nine innings without allowing a single runner on base. Perfection conjures up images of harder-to-define conditions too, like the "perfect" body, "perfect" health, "perfect" mate, even the "perfect" life as viewed through the lens of social media.

Research suggests that our pursuit of perfection has risen significantly in recent years as part of a major ideological shift at a societal level. Many have become beleaguered by the need to reach what, in most cases, is an unattainable preordained ideal. Even when we do achieve our definition of perfection, we become obsessed with the idea of upping the ante, getting caught on a treadmill of ceaseless yearning and perpetual dissatisfaction. Unsurprisingly, studies show that the desire for perfection is often a burden and a major source of unhappiness. In our pursuit of it, contentment is constrained and joy bridled.

The kind of perfection I discuss in this book is different. It bears closer resemblance to a concept of perfection that dates back to antiquity—the idea that perfection can only be found in imperfection and that growth, progress, and the assembly of imperfect factors make perfection possible.

One could compare it to the weather. A "perfect" day involves a pleasant coming together of temperature, wind speed, sunlight, and the like. Change any one of those independent factors and the perfect day might not materialize; and what constitutes a perfect day for one person won't for another. Indeed, the perception of perfection can even be influenced by what came before it—a hot, muggy day that makes way for a "perfectly" cool, sunny tomorrow.

Importantly, while you have the agency to set yourself up to enjoy what might turn into what you perceive to be a perfect day, you can't will it into existence. You have no control over the jet stream, wind speed, or movement of the sun. But you can be present and well positioned to bask in it when it arises.

The "perfect run," as I describe it in this book, is much the same way. It develops spontaneously, coalescing body, mind, and spirit in an enigmatic way that can only be described as perfection. It arises in the presence of an acceptance of the imperfect and mysterious nature of the factors that convene to produce the state. So often we seek perfection through control, but it's in the letting go that true perfection ensues. Consider my run through the mountains of Big Sky: Leading up to the race, I hadn't been doing any altitude training and my mind was more focused on parenting than running. But once the elk horn sounded, I released any expectations and allowed myself to exist in the moment. That's when a number of seemingly imperfect elements came together to elicit a perfect run.

In my definition, the "perfect run" encompasses a variety of experiences, from bursts of power and endurance to feelings of effortlessness and oneness, to sensations of levity and euphoria. Runners of every experience and competitive level describe feeling in complete control, a reverberation of the senses, a surge of energy, a hyperfocus, a mental and physical synchronicity, and a total immersion in the moment.

Exercise physiologist and coach Greg McMillan put it to me this way: "It's a feeling that is hard to define or explain to someone who hasn't experienced it. Your focus narrows and you feel a sense of great contentment, even though you're pushing your body. It's a place where you enjoy and relish in the challenge of the run. There's this feeling of 'man, I wish I could live in that more often.'"

Having experienced these types of runs many times over my 25 years of running, I've long been interested in the concept of "the perfect run." For much of that time, however, I struggled to achieve them with any consistency. Sometimes they'd materialize in the midst of a great training cycle when everything was going according to plan. But I've also slipped into that special state following some of the worst runs of my life when I was on the verge of quitting and hanging up my kicks for good.

As it turns out, this is a phenomenon that can be harnessed to some degree. While it can't be forced, research suggests that the stage can be purposefully set for the perfect running state to arise more readily. In my quest to understand this perfect running headspace, I started with a basic level of understanding based on my experience as a running journalist and coach and my academic background in sports psychology. As I dug further into the research and spoke with coaches, psychologists, physiologists, and neuroscientists, as well as surveying professional and recreational runners, I soon found that I was generating more questions than answers. I wanted to know: What are the psychological conditions that prompt the perfect running experience? What prevents it? What outside factors might contribute to or detract from it? Why does the experience feel like it occurs with varying levels of intensity? Is there a way to call it up on command?

This book garners research from both on and off the running trails, revealing important lessons about how to conjure these perfect runs. Positioning your body and mind to achieve more perfect running experiences requires knowledge, practice, and patience. There's no blueprint or predetermined steps you take to get there, but rather a set of principles that may help you find it. And while the perfect running state can certainly be a boon to performance, you'll notice that my focus remains on enhancing the running experience. Healthier training, improved fitness, and better performance are by-products.

These types of optimal experiences are said to be a centerpiece of a satisfying life, and running—for elite athletes and recreational

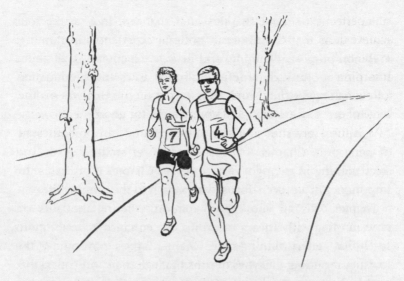

Fulfillment in running and life can go hand in hand.

runners alike—just happens to be one very apt place to discover them. Research shows that the more fulfillment people tend to experience in life, the more activities in which they also encounter what I call perfection. To be sure, there is a reciprocal relationship at play—this state of perfection, when one is immersed in the run and enjoying the activity in the moment for its own sake—also feeds that sense of fulfillment. Rather than finding happiness in an end goal or future pay-off, research suggests that the seeds of joy in life are sown through remaining present along each chapter— or mile—of the journey. Hopefully by learning to harness more perfect runs, you'll be better able to reach this transcendent headspace in other areas of life as well.

In Chapter 1, we'll look at the anatomy of the perfect run and break down what these experiences look and feel like. While much about this state remains a mystery, thanks to a wealth of recent scientific research there's much we have come to understand. Chapter 2 will make the case for running as a vehicle into this state. The next several chapters after that will look at the four main factors that contribute to optimal experiences in running: Presence, purpose, planning, and process. Chapter 3 is all about how presence through mindfulness builds an essential foundation for cultivating the right conditions for perfect running experiences. In Chapter 4, we'll look at how developing an authentic sense of purpose serves as a major driver toward this special state of perfection. Chapter 5 covers how to set strategic goals and steer training in the right direction and Chapter 6 discusses the importance of a process-focused approach to the running life.

Chapter 7 is all about participation, offering thoughts on how running with a team or group can enhance your ability to reach that perfect running state. Chapter 8 goes into some of the logistics regarding the types of runs that can transport you to that next-level headspace. Finally, Chapter 9 includes advice on what to do when you've lost your running mojo and perfect running feels all but out of reach.

The Perfect Run recounts the stories I've collected during my research, as well as discoveries I've made along the path of my own running journey. I will discuss the transformational power of running and what finding transcendence on the run can teach us about living a good and fulfilling life. These powerful moments of presence, when you feel like a conduit for the energy of the universe, offer glimpses of a special variety of perfection. Best of all, they are accessible to runners of every level and pace. Through first-hand narratives and hands-on exercises, the coming pages will demonstrate how to make the leap from theory to practice, ensuring a more joyful experience not only as you navigate the running trails, but also well beyond.

Chapter 1
DISCOVERING PERFECTION

*"Instead of driving to a perfect surface to run, I was
allowing myself to go where my heart went, where my
legs took me. And I began to reconnect with my deep,
deep, deep love for the sport, and what it means to me."*

ON A MUGGY, 80-degree (27°C) evening in late June, I crouched
trackside near the finish line on the first night of the 2008 U.S.
Olympic trials for track and field. Amid a throng of photographers
and reporters, I worked to get a good angle on the competition.
The setting sun made way for a pink, dusky hue, encapsulating
the stadium grounds. Eight tall light poles surrounding the all-
weather track flickered on to illuminate Hayward Field. The
spotlight event of the evening—the women's 10,000 meters—was
lining up. This opening final of the ten-day trials would determine
U.S. track and field's first 2008 Olympians. The athletes and their
nearly 21,000 fans glowed with an anticipation that hung in the
sultry summer air.

Over 1,000 athletes, 1,200 visiting media, and 167,000 fans
from around the world descended on the town of Eugene,
Oregon, which was normally home to just 150,000 people. Sitting
at an elevation of 400 feet (122 meters), the town is nestled in
the Willamette Valley between the Pacific Ocean and Cascade
Mountain Range. The area is known for its green landscape marked

by tall trees, winding natural footpaths, and the Willamette River. At the heart of Eugene is the University of Oregon campus where the legendary Hayward Field is located.

Known as Tracktown, USA, it has been host to countless U.S. Olympic trials, national championships, and other big track and field events over the decades. It was here at Hayward Field in the 1960s that Oregon coach Bill Bowerman introduced the sport of running to the masses to spark the American "jogging" craze, giving birth to the Nike brand. The charismatic Steve Prefontaine simultaneously elevated himself and Hayward Field to legendary status during his time at the University of Oregon. The 1972 Olympian would set American records in the 2,000 meters all the way through the 10,000 meters. At the age of 25 he was tragically killed in a car accident just a mile or so from the oval.

At 9:20 p.m. Pacific Standard Time, the gun fired, signaling the start of the women's 10,000-meter race. The 25-lap race featured a duel between the 2007 World Championship bronze medalist,

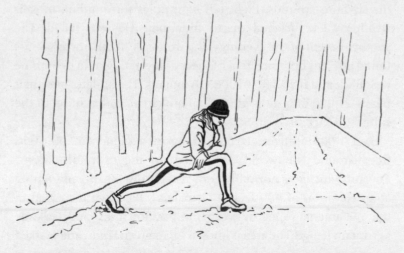

Perfection can be found in the heat of competition or on a solitary jog.

Kara Goucher, and the American record holder in the 10,000, Shalane Flanagan. The race got off to a fast pace with the two best hopes for American distance-running medals battling it out stride for stride.

By the halfway point, the pair, along with Goucher's training partner, Amy Yoder Begley, broke away from the larger pack. Yoder Begley pushed from the front for the majority of the last 3,000 meters of the race before trading spots with Goucher, Flanagan running in third. With 1,200 meters remaining, Goucher and Flanagan surged ahead. Every move Flanagan made, Goucher countered, but with 300 meters to go, the American record holder made one final decisive push to capture first place ahead of Goucher and Yoder Begley.

Shortly after, I gathered with other reporters under a stuffy white tent for the post-race press conference. Goucher was thrilled to have punched her ticket to the Olympics, but wondered aloud why she hadn't pushed harder on the homestretch. "I feel like I gave up a little on the last lap," she said.

Six days later I was trackside again to watch her line up against Flanagan for another warm nighttime race—the 5,000-meter final. While they got off to a slower start, with 1,200 meters to go the gloves came off and Flanagan surged, bringing two-time Olympian Jen Rhines and Goucher with her. Goucher bided her time in third place for most of the race, but in the last 200 meters, as the trio came around the final curve, she kicked hard. Lengthening her stride and pumping her arms, she first passed Rhines and then Flanagan for a blazing fast 4:36 final mile and a first-place finish. Later in the press conference she would say, "With 200 to go … it was one of those moments … I just had to risk it."

From my vantage point down at the finish line, I alternated between viewing Goucher on the big screen and watching her live on the track as she sailed by every 400 meters. There was a distinct resoluteness to her execution in the final laps of that race. Something clicked. Her stride looked fluid and strong. She leaned into each step with precision. Her confidence clearly soared.

Recently Goucher told me this: "Sometimes you hit this flow and the hard session or race you are running just streams on by. It's not that it isn't hard—it still is—but there is a joy in being in control of your body and being able to push it along the edge. Honestly, one of my favorite feelings in the world is riding that line. Pushing myself so hard, but holding back just a hair, knowing that if I push any more, I will blow up and my lungs will burst. It's such a great feeling."

She would go on to finish eighth in the 5,000 meters and tenth in the 10,000 meters in Beijing. The next Olympic cycle she earned a spot on the U.S. Olympic marathon squad, where she finished eleventh. She became one of the country's most successful distance runners and firmly affixed herself in the running history books. But after more than a decade spent at the top with countless encounters with perfect running like that day in Eugene, she began to reexamine her career. She found herself looking for renewed joy and meaning in her running— a different kind of perfection that was more reminiscent of the type that characterized her early years in the sport as a youngster.

She ended up finding it in 2017 on a gravel road in Northern Minnesota near her mother's home. A far cry from the impeccably groomed trails and manicured tracks where she normally trained, she navigated each step over and around rutted-out potholes, deep-set tire tracks, jagged rocks, and precarious patches of grit. She first discovered a passion for running on these roads when she was 12 years old. She wrote about that day in an essay for the website Motiv: "Instead of driving to a perfect surface to run, I was allowing myself to go where my heart went, where my legs took me. And I began to reconnect with my deep, deep, deep love for the sport, and what it means to me."

In recalling that run, she later told me, "It made me feel free and full of joy. I loved running through nature and running just to run. Over time I became more focused on competition and with how much I could get out of myself every day. I don't regret chasing my career with all I had, but it's nice to get back to the freedom of just loving the experience for what it is. For feeling free to move in a way I love."

It was a different kind of perfect run she encountered that day on that secluded road in the Northwoods, but equally momentous as the flowy runs she's experienced on the national and world stages. She contends that running perfection comes in varying intensities and that sticking with the sport through the highs and lows is essential. She added: "You just need to get out there and run. Sometimes you are building fitness or in a slump and you won't feel it for ages. And then it will come, unexpectedly. You'll be out on a long run and you'll see the miles are just coming and coming and you are on the edge, but the right side of the edge. Just get out there and you will find it. It takes time but eventually you will have one of those days."

***

A Brief History of Perfection

Goucher hints at the fact that while perfect runs occur on a spectrum, they all have the potential to influence your running in important ways. The emergence of research on optimal experiences came in the 1970s when Hungarian psychologist Mihaly Csikszentmihalyi coined the term "flow" to define a "highly focused state of consciousness." Interest in how enjoyment and satisfaction were cultivated led him to interview a wide demographic: Artists, surgeons, rock climbers, farmers, parents, chess-masters, and assembly-line workers, among others. Interestingly, they all described the feeling of performing at their best and being totally engrossed in an activity in similar terms. Whether they were harvesting fields, meditating, or performing open-heart surgery, the people he interviewed all shared a feeling of optimal consciousness.

These types of experiences have been referenced in various cultures and traditions in a myriad of ways. In Japan, "Shibumi" is a Zen concept that roughly describes something similar to flow and is often referenced as "effortless perfection." Likewise, yogis will recognize many of the components of flow as sharing similarities with Sage Patanjali's eightfold path described in ancient texts that were written around 400 CE.

Some have spoken of "optimal" and "transcendent" experiences and say they offer an encounter with nirvana. Others prefer less religious connotations to describe this phenomenon. Back in the early 1960s, novelist and professed atheist Marghanita Laski conducted a widely cited survey on these types of encounters with the mystical, opting for the term "ecstatic experiences." More recently, environmental psychologist Louise Chawla also referred to them as "ecstatic" moments. Fittingly, in Greek, the word "ecstasy" means to "stand outside oneself."

In their 1978 book, *In the Zone*, Michael Murphy and Rhea White extensively chronicled transcendent experiences in sport, labeling them as "metanormal" and "extraordinary," and representing a level of human functioning that far exceeds the typical. It is also often noted that the descriptions of optimal experience share many characteristics with observations made by famed American psychologist Abraham Maslow in his research investigating the lives of people who exemplified top human performance. He sought commonalities between these individuals in hopes of cracking the code on human achievement and the accompanying sense of self-transcendence. He described them as "peak experiences," labeling them "mystic and magical."

There is no shortage of descriptions in the literature that refer specifically to running as well, all of which I classify under the umbrella of "perfect running experiences." For instance, famous French explorer and Buddhist Madame Alexandra David-Neel reported three separate encounters with the legendary "lung-gom-pa runners" during her 14 years spent living in Tibet in the early 1900s. According to lore, they could run days at a time and cover upward of 200 miles (320 km) in a single 24-hour period. In her book *Magic and Mystery in Tibet*, David-Neel wrote of the calm, seemingly effortless manner of running the lung-gom-pa runners achieved—describing it as meditative and almost trance-like. She insisted that it wasn't physical strength that made them capable of these extraordinary feats of endurance, but training resulting in "psychic states."

In his study of runners, renowned psychiatrist and author Dr. William Glasser described it as a transcendental mindset, similar to that reached by monks. It has been suggested that the running rhythm has a natural way of lifting a person beyond oneself toward a state of exaltation, even comparing it to repetition in other activities, like "om" in meditation or "Hail Mary" in Catholic traditions. To be sure, that encounter with perfection feels spiritual to many runners. One study found that nearly half of the runners surveyed experienced a running-induced euphoria that they defined as spiritual in nature.

After spending two years traveling to different countries talking to runners about their experiences, Finnish runner and researcher Noora Ronkainen reported that many runners identified existential meaning and a spiritual connection to the sport thanks to optimal experiences. Inspired by the writings of Catholic theologian Karl Rahner, who discussed how spirituality could be revealed in daily life, she wrote:

> *"Fascinated with the idea of encountering the sacred in everyday activities, I reflected upon it in my running. I became aware of how some of my runs were moments of strong presence. When running, I sensed myself and the beauty of my surroundings in dimensions not accessible during other events in my everyday living, such as a tram trip across the city. Through my running I started to discover what Rahner (1979) meant by the spiritual in the ordinary, and our blindness to the sacred and mystical in our everyday lives."*

Physician, author, and preeminent running philosopher Dr. George Sheehan simply called this experience the "third wind" to describe the feeling of everything coming together on a run at just the right time. The first sub-four-minute miler, Sir Roger Bannister, portrayed it as a "great unity of movement."

When I surveyed everyday runners about their perfect running experiences, they told me things like: "I feel relaxed and don't have pain," "It's running euphoria, I feel indestructible, like I could run over a mountain and not get winded," "It's easeful and exhilarating all at the same time," "I feel calm, effortless, and timeless," "I feel strong, smooth and confident," "I'm entirely in the moment," and "It's completely an ethereal sense of oneness between body, soul, and the universe."

One of my favorite descriptions came from professional ultrarunner Michael Wardian in early 2019, soon after he shattered the record for the fastest completion of ten marathons in ten consecutive days, seven of which were run on seven different continents. He told me this:

> *"I would describe it as an effortless kinetic sensory experience unaffected by time, gravity, and circumstance.*

When I reach this state on a run I feel empowered, full, complete, confident, and each step is effortless. I am smooth, fluid, my mind clears, and I know this is what I am meant to do. I feel content, at home, and fulfilled. I am not cold, or hot or tired, or hungry or amped. I just am. Some might think it is Zen-like, but I just feel bliss."

Perhaps the most common term runners recognize to describe these types of experiences is "the runner's high." Research out of Florida State University found that a full 77 percent of runners they surveyed said they'd experienced it first-hand. Sharing much in common with flow, the term was originally coined when runners' descriptions of the state mirrored those of drug-induced highs. In the literature, no clear definition exists. One study noted at least 27 different adjectives that are used to describe it, including euphoria, strength, speed, and spirituality. Most often it is characterized by feelings of exaltation, joy, relaxation, and decreased anxiety and pain.

While the runner's high is a chemical response to running, flow is a bit more complicated, involving psychological and situational precursors that generally go hand in hand with optimal performance. Neuroscientist Leslie Sherlin, who has run more than 20 marathons and is the co-founder of a San Francisco-based purveyor of brain training research, put it to me this way:

"In the flow state, you're having timeless moments where effort and challenge balance and you're able to perform in ways that are beyond your typical ability. Whereas runner's high can happen more easily. It shares those feelings of euphoria with flow, but doesn't necessarily involve those aspects of having challenge present or enhanced performance. As an illustration, you could experience a runner's high when you go out for a run and the weather is nice, you're really present, you're enjoying

the moment, your body is engaged and just feeling really good. That's different than when you go out and push your body to new levels, running slightly outside of your normal capacity and you fall into that flow experience where performance is beyond the effort and ability you previously demonstrated. That enhanced performance attribute and higher level of pushing yourself is the differentiator."

To be sure, the perfect running state is not an on/off switch, but rather an experience that occurs in varying intensities. Consider a couple of examples:

Perhaps you've been training for a 5K race for months and as soon as the gun fires, you take off and everything clicks. You feel totally engaged and in control as you push your body to its limits. Time telescopes, then falls away. Minutes feel like seconds. A transcendence takes hold as you perform and feel at your very best. That's a perfect run.

As Sherlin suggested, perfect running can also occur in lesser intensities in the most ordinary of circumstances on everyday training runs. Maybe it's the first warm day of spring and you head out for a moderately paced 4-miler (6.5-km). The sun is out, the birds are chirping, and your legs feel fresh. Partway into the run, you become completely absorbed in the experience. Your mood lifts to the point of elation and you have the sensation that you could run forever. That's a perfect run too.

It is important to note that although the runner's high is thought to be more easily accessible, those feelings of exaltation and euphoria can play a major role in motivating a runner to continue to train, which thereby may lead to the deeper flow state. While distinctions exist between these terms, keep in mind that even those who have devoted their careers to studying these phenomena don't completely understand them. Semantics aside, throughout this book I will reference these optimal experiences as all falling under the canopy of "perfect running." In the simplest terms, when you achieve a "perfect" run, you enter a superfluid state where mood is elevated and actions flow. You are so focused on the run that everything else fades into the background. Your sense of time and self disappear and you experience a merging of action and awareness. Transcendence and joy follow. Importantly, this experience is accessible to runners of all backgrounds, ambitions, and experience levels.

What runners say

I surveyed everyday runners to get a better handle on the range and intensity of perfect running experiences. Here's what they had to say:

"As a long-time runner, I've found myself in the flow state many times. I feel chills and the hair on the back of my neck might even stand up. It's running euphoria and I feel indestructible, like I could run over a mountain and not get winded."

John G., 40, Philadelphia, PA

"I experience this feeling often. It occurs when I'm both fit and rested. Lack of fitness and/or tiredness and fatigue precludes the feeling of being in the zone."

Tom D., 58, Sydney, Australia

"An instance of being 'in the zone' that stands out the most for me was a trail run on a beautiful September day in Colorado. The aspens were at peak gold levels, there was a creek running alongside the trail and we were going straight up 1,200 feet in the first two miles. The first mile I cursed myself for proposing this run, but once my legs started to wake up, I realized I was just focusing on each step and it became almost meditative. I was hearing the creek and my breath, feeling the breeze and every muscle in my legs working, and just going step by step. Then suddenly, we hit the top of the climb and I just flew downhill through the aspens from there."

Meg S., 29, Denver, CO

"Physically and mentally it feels as though your body is in complete harmony with running, you are running at the perfect speed, you don't feel tired physically, and nothing is hurting. In your head, you feel invincible, like you could run forever at a decent speed."

Sarah E., 49, Hereford, UK

"My feet were flying effortlessly on the trail. The single track was not smooth but I had total confidence that there were going to be no disasters. My nearest competitor was beating me on the uphills, but my turnover was so smooth on the downhill and I knew I would ultimately prevail. The weather was horrendous—pouring rain and windy—but that only increased the pure joy."

Reesie K., 44, San Jose, CA

"It felt like I could push the pace with no extra strain—not that I could go infinitely faster, but I was very sure of my ability to perform and run a certain pace. I was very much in the moment, but not so much so that I lost the big picture of how much work there was left to do."

Nikki D., 36, Frisco, TX

"I feel in the flow of a run when I'm moving with ease, enjoying myself, and coping confidently with whatever the weather and terrain throw at me."

Phil B., 55, Basingstoke, Hampshire, UK

"I wasn't distracted by anything—just totally focused on executing the race. The discomfort was not overwhelming, despite it being very high. For some reason, it's like I just didn't care that I was hurting. All I wanted was more: More speed, more pain, and more hammering."

Jason F., 35, Denver, CO

"Physically I felt like running was effortless and I was running much faster than normal, like I almost could not hold back the speed. Everything was in sync—form, breathing, focus. Psychologically I felt very positive, almost a state of joy. I have been known to smile the times this has happened. There is also a wistfulness, because you know it won't last, so I really try to enjoy it in the moment."

Ken H., 58, Manteca, CA

***

The Anatomy of a Perfect Run

To better pin down what a perfect run actually looks and feels like, we'll dive deeper into the neuroscience involved, as well as more observational anecdotes gathered by experts. I will also draw upon descriptions of the perfect running state made to me directly by coaches, neuroscientists, and professional and recreational runners.

The Neuroscience

While experts are far from fully understanding exactly what is going on in the brain when we enter this elevated state on a run, they have plenty of theories. There is still much to be discovered about the way thoughts and emotions travel along the hills and valleys of our brain's inner circuitry. What we do know is that when the perfect running experience arises, a complicated combination of electrical, chemical, and architectural components are at work.

Electrical

At the center of some of the most exciting new research on flow is the study of brain wave activity. Neurons are constantly communicating with each other and sending out synchronized electrical pulses across the brain. This activity changes depending on what you're doing—when a run becomes more challenging, for instance, specific brain waves are activated. Brain waves occur at different frequencies and in different patterns depending on what the brain is doing—making decisions, pondering creative insights, willing your body to push harder at the end of a race, or resting.

From fastest to slowest, the following are the five types of brain waves:

- **Gamma** These waves are associated with higher processing activities, in particular recognized for "ah ha!" moments. These waves are active when the parts of the brain are working together to bind thoughts.
- **Beta** These waves are involved with paying attention, reasoning, and problem-solving.
- **Alpha** These waves are usually active when you're relaxed and thoughts are flowing effortlessly. You're lucid, but your brain is at rest. This is often referred to as "idling."
- **Theta** These waves are associated with daydreaming and light sleep.
- **Delta** These waves are involved in deep sleep.

Sherlin, the neuroscientist I previously mentioned, has worked with over 1,300 high performers, including professional athletes, musicians, and top executives, to examine the EEG signatures involved when someone is functioning at a high level. Although tracking their brain activity while in flow is tricky, especially for athletes who must be in motion to achieve the state, Sherlin has some ideas about what is going on in the brain.

"We theorize that there is a decrease in faster frequency activity—so diminished beta—and an increase of alpha in certain regions of the brain," he explained. "Gamma bursts happen whenever we have eureka experiences and we go 'ah ha!' So it would be natural for those waves to be present in flow state too—but they aren't likely to last long as we are quickly back in the experience."

Many runners will begin a run in beta—you're thinking about the details of the workout, what you'll have for dinner, and the day's to-do list. Research suggests that you can cross into the flow state around the border of alpha and theta, which is the line between the conscious and subconscious mind and the point at which that mental yammering ceases and you exist totally in the moment. There's still much to be learned in this field, but one thing most everyone agrees on is that there is a clear shift in activity in a number of different areas of the brain.

Chemical

For decades, experts have pondered what neurochemicals might be involved in optimal experiences. While we don't completely understand how, when, and which chemicals are released into the bloodstream during a perfect run, we do know they play a role in transmitting messages throughout the brain and influencing this state of mind. "The neurochemicals modulate the electricity in the brain, so the fact that we can see a shift in electrical patterns also means there's a shift in neurotransmitters," explains Sherlin.

Some of the neurochemicals thought to be potentially involved include endocannabinoids, endorphins, dopamine, norepinephrine, serotonin, GABA, and adrenaline. Evolutionarily speaking, some research even suggests that the release of these chemicals is what helped transform humans into long-distance runners—a skill of persistence that we relied upon to chase down prey. As the research on the brain chemistry involved in these states continues to evolve, surely so too will the theories regarding which neurochemical mechanisms are at work.

Architectural

On top of the electrical and chemical fluctuations that occur when you reach that special brain state on a perfect run, there are thought to be changes in brain structures and neural networks. Even back in the 1980s, psychiatrist William Glasser, M.D., theorized that in this state the brain is freed up to create new neural networks, allowing novel pathways to form and the brain to grow in important ways.

One of the most recent theories, posited by neuroscientist Arne Dietrich, PhD., is known as Transient Hypofrontality. "Transient" means temporary and "hypofrontality" is a reference to the slowing down of the prefrontal cortex. The idea behind the Transient Hypofrontality Theory is that, as the demands of a task increase, the brain reduces the energy it offers to nonessential functions. For instance, the prefrontal cortex downregulates in order to simply process basic information.

Sherlin explains it this way: "Your prefrontal cortex is this planning and organization center that decides what to do or say next depending on the task you're involved in. When there is decreased activation, it goes into this monitoring state where you're not planning the next moment from a cognitive standpoint. Things are happening in a way that are not premeditated. The way flow has been described, it is this moment of mastery and acceptance and not having to analyze what you're going to do next."

Observational Research

While the neuroscience is still in the nascent phases, there is much observational and self-reported evidence surrounding optimal experiences. In particular, Csikszentmihalyi has worked to define the specific elements that characterize the flow state. In my research, I discovered much crossover with descriptors of the perfect running state. As I described in the introduction, these experiences are akin to the weather. No single element measures or dictates it, but there are several factors that contribute to it that can be measured and analyzed. While not all of the following characteristics need be present to achieve a perfect run, the research suggests at least some will be involved.

Unshakeable focus

A supreme level of concentration is a hallmark of the perfect running state. Kim Conley, a two-time U.S. Olympian in the 5,000 meters, told me this: "I've found that I best achieve running in the zone during a race or workout when I allow myself to be fully immersed in the moment. Instead of thinking ahead to what I want to do or how I want to feel later in the race, I try to stay present with what is unfolding in that moment. When I can zone in on the present, I have an easier time blocking out external distractions, maintaining engagement, and generally feeling like I am in the flow of the race."

As Conley asserts, when you're totally absorbed in the run, your attentional energy is focused on the most relevant stimuli. This means you aren't worried about your tired legs or the weather or the pile of laundry you have to take care of when you get home. Rather, you are switched on and able to sift out extraneous data that may threaten to interrupt the flow of the run so you can focus on pertinent information, like your pace or how your legs feel.

Universal oneness

When you achieve this level of focus, you are "one" with the run. A normally challenging effort feels effortless and you fall into a rhythm despite great physical output. You are so immersed in the run that body and mind work in perfect synchrony.

When I asked 10,000-meter Greek-American Olympian Alexi Pappas about this, she replied, "When I'm running and my mind and body are on the same page, it feels like I am in complete harmony with myself. It's a very special feeling."

Total control

While we often carry the vague dread that we aren't in complete control in many areas of our lives, a compelling sense of confidence and jurisdiction constitute a perfect run. Mohammed Ahmed, two-time Canadian Olympian, put it to me this way: "When I am in the zone, there is a control and confidence. It's a worry-free state, an ability to speed up and slow down at the drop of a dime, read a situation in seemingly slow-motion state, and to visualize things before they have fully developed. It's a state where you feel like you can't be stopped and where things are done instinctually or intuitively with fluidity and laser focus."

As Ahmed asserts, in this state you feel calm, composed, and even empowered. It's as if one good move makes way for another and another, like doors are automatically opening ahead of you. While some outside force could impede your control—a sudden rainstorm or an aggressive competitor—this state offers a brief sense of invincibility that is challenging to harness elsewhere.

Egoless awareness

When you're in a perfect run, self-conscious thoughts fall away. You don't devote energy to petty self-judgment or evaluation; rather, you simply let your body run. While you're aware of your sphere of consciousness, unproductive thoughts that often weigh you down disappear. It is a liberation from anxieties, doubts, and insecurities.

Irish Olympian in the marathon, Paul Pollock, describes this by saying, "It's a quasi self-hypnotic state. All external stimuli become meaningless, going unnoticed. Pain seems unable to touch you. Everything remains relaxed and your one goal resonates repeatedly in your mind, 'Let's just keep this going.' Thoughts seem to cease. You aren't worried. You do not feel pressure. Even time itself seems to have no bearing on your world."

Modified sense of time
It is on those perfect runs when hours can feel like minutes and minutes like seconds—the natural ebb and flow of your day simply melts away. You exist in an almost timeless state where your perception of the passage of time is altered. It doesn't mean that you aren't keeping track of pace or splits, but that the actual feeling of time becomes an abstraction.

Angie Petty, a 2016 Olympic 800-meter runner from New Zealand, explains it by saying, "I think in the flow state you are just very focused on what you are doing and block out all distractions. Time seems to pass at a different speed, slower in a way, but then also really fast."

Intrinsic joy
The result of these other components is a marked sense of joy. It's not about your fitness or the accolades, but the in-the-moment

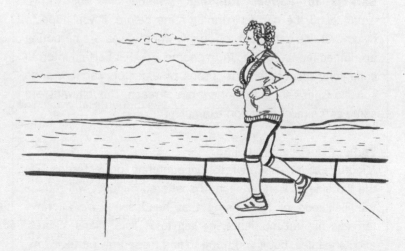

A number of factors come together to elicit a perfect run.

experience of running. To be sure, for the perfect running experience to arise in the first place, a love of the sport must exist on some level.

As Deena Kastor told me: "If you practice going into workouts and races with calm excitement and a sense of gratitude, not only will you have a healthier mindset, it also creates a chemical reaction in your body, which allows you to get the most out of a run or race. In the end, the goal in and of itself should be to achieve joy."

Reaching that perfect state of mind on the run will further develop your passion for running. This is an entirely unique experience because with many things, we do them out of obligation or hopes of pay-off down the road. The intrinsic satisfaction of a flowy run allows you to exist and feel fulfilled in the moment. While experts are still working to fully understand these types of optimal experiences, anecdotal evidence points to the fact that running is a great place to find it. The following chapter will dive into why running offers such an ideal platform for perfection to arise.

Barriers to Perfect Running: Whether or not you've experienced the perfect running state before, if you hope to discover it, it's important to identify whether you are harboring any impediments to flow. In the same way that certain internal conditions encourage perfect runs, other factors can rearrange consciousness so as to make it out of reach. The following are some of the most common examples.

Barrier #1: A Scattered Mind
Mindfulness is essential to encountering perfect runs. On the flip side, a wandering and scattered mindset will reduce the likelihood of harnessing that headspace. We all have tornadic mental moments, cycling to-do lists, plans, chores, and schedules, but if you hope to find those truly perfect runs,

---

you must learn to establish the mental discipline to focus on the task at hand when you're running. Research shows that learning to control your attentional energy and focus on the task directly in front of you boosts enjoyment of the activity and sows the seeds of flow. We'll learn more about the benefits of mindfulness in Chapter 3.

Barrier #2: Stress and Anxiety

Stress and anxiety are realities of modern existence and can't simply be eliminated at the drop of a hat. With that said, if you hope to find flow, it is important to muster the attentional willpower to shelve stress in order to focus on your run. In my experience, this can take a mile or two of intentional concentration on the run before I fall into the rhythm of movement and at least momentarily let my worries fade into the background of my consciousness.

Keep in mind that if your stress and anxiety is related to running itself, you should step back and reevaluate your running goals and training as a whole. While a calculated amount of stress—say the nerves associated with taking on a big goal—might help nurture flow, too much stress inhibits it. In fact, several researchers have noted that an overly competitive environment or mindset is a sure way to kill the chances of reaching this state of mind. This is largely because competition can involve self-judgment and endless evaluation, distracting from the simple rhythm of running. If you're feeling the weight of internal or external pressures and expectations, finding joy and equanimity in your running life will prove difficult. These topics will be touched upon further in Chapters 4 and 5, but let this be your first nudge to reexamine the course of your training if it's causing stress in your life.

Barrier #3: Running Insecurities

Possibly connected to stress and anxiety, if you're overly self-conscious or wrapped up in constant self-judgment, you may find it particularly challenging to achieve that next-level headspace on the run. This could be related to worries about the way you look when you run or how your finishing time will be perceived by others. Not only do these things make it difficult to enjoy almost anything you do, it signals a lack of control in your attentional energy. The constant distraction of self-evaluation will make it all but impossible to fully focus on the run at hand. We all have our moments of self-criticism, but finding ways to discipline the mind to focus on more productive thinking is essential to discovering those perfect runs. I'll go into this in greater detail in Chapter 4.

Barrier #4: A Negative Attitude

Training will never be all rainbows and unicorns every time you slip on your running shoes. We all have days when we are tired or rushed and running is the last thing we want to do. With that said, your overall outlook on running should trend positive. If you find that negativity is clouding your mind during your runs, you'll have trouble finding anything that resembles perfect running. More importantly, this attitude may signal that you need to take some sort of action. In addition to a whole host of physical symptoms, looming negativity of mind goes hand in hand with overtraining and burnout. If you're less than enthusiastic about running on a regular basis, it may be time to lay off of pounding the pavement to give your body and mind a break. I'll address this further in Chapter 9.

Barrier #5: Boredom

Novelty is essential when it comes to perfect running experiences. If you run the same route at the same pace and distance day after day, it's easy to become complacent. Boredom encourages the mind to wander away from what is going on in the moment in search of something more interesting. New challenges or scenery have a way of waking up the mind to the joys of running. If you're in a funk when it comes to your training practices, consider mixing things up. The topic of boredom will be addressed in Chapters 5 and 9.

Barrier #6: Environmental Concerns
This is an obvious one. If you don't feel safe in your environment, for whatever reason, you won't be able to achieve that perfect running state. Whether it's due to personal safety, weather, or some other factor, safety should be your number one concern when heading out on a run.

Practices in Perfection

- Optimal experiences come in many shapes, sizes, and levels of intensity.
- "Perfect running experiences" exist on a spectrum, encompassing a variety of terms, including "flow," the "runner's high," and the "zone."
- While we don't fully understand the neural mechanisms that are involved in these optimal states of consciousness, it is theorized that electrical, chemical, and architectural components are at work.
- Perfect runs share a number of characteristics: Unshakeable focus, universal oneness, total control, egoless awareness, modified sense of time, and intrinsic joy.

Chapter 2

RUNNING AS A TRAINING GROUND FOR PERFECTION

*"I get up, carry on running and laugh aloud to myself.
I'm feeling a bit crazy. Am I losing it? I don't give
a damn. I lose control again and slip down into a
muddy hollow. This is life. I'm completely consumed
by nature."*

MARKUS TORGEBY TAKES off first at a walk, soon picking up the pace and running toward Lake Helgesjön. He can't resist the impulse to move freely through the deep wilderness in one of the coldest and most isolated regions of northern Sweden. He stumbles through spongy marshes, ducks under branches, and splashes through small streams that are beginning to feel icy with the autumn air. The forest has seeded itself so completely that the looming fir and birch stand dense and tall around him. He takes in the earthy smells created by the chemicals released from eons of growth and decomposition. The sun is high in the sky and the clouds crawl over the peaks of Åreskutan mountain 9 miles (15 km) in the distance, already covered in snow.

Torgeby hasn't seen another human being in over three weeks. His back and arms ache from chopping firewood to build up his supply for the long winter in the woods. His body is weary but content from sleeping on a horsehair mattress in his self-made canvas-covered teepee and subsisting on porridge, berries, nuts, and birch sap. "I have never spent so much time on my own," he wrote in his bestselling memoir *The Runner*. "It feels strange. Time moves more slowly. I breathe more deeply, and I can feel my heart beating."

Between the ages of 20 and 24, Torgeby lived alone in the woods, only making periodic trips to visit civilization. Each day, he wrote, "I get up, I eat, I run, I try not to freeze." Born in 1976 in Öckerö, an island off the western coast of Sweden that is part of the Northern Gothenburg Archipelago, he was identified as a top-tier talent on the track as a youngster. In the beginning, running provided him a sense of freedom and an escape from the stress involved with caring for his mother, who had been diagnosed with multiple sclerosis. Over time, however, the pressure to compete led to overtraining and burnout. What was once his passion led to a string of injuries and persistent feelings of restlessness.

Without running as a refuge, and overwhelmed by his stressful home life, he made a dramatic move: He bought himself a one-way train ticket, rode it as far north as he could go, and walked into the

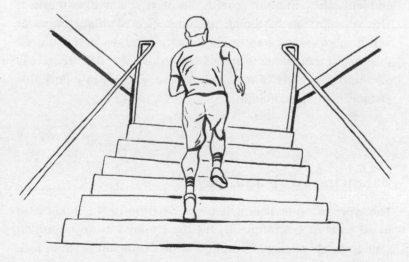

Embracing running as more than a competitive endeavor is essential to reaching that special state of perfection.

woods 30 or so miles (48 km) with a rucksack on his back carrying clothes, food, and equipment. Over time he constructed a shelter and adopted a solitary routine. Each day he woke to run, moving until he was soaked to the skin, or his legs were tired, or darkness fell. He hunted, fished, and foraged for berries, cooked over an open fire, and fell asleep watching the moon through a hole in his teepee. He learned that in the forest, he could simply focus on survival. The stress lifted and body, mind, and spirit fell into sync. He wrote:

"I disappeared into myself, the outside world vanished ... Everything was clear: My head, the air, my thoughts ... My brain is whirring nicely, I'm tired, happy and seriously hungry. I lie down on the bed. I don't think about anything at all. I don't feel any longing for anything at all. I am completely content."

Torgeby rediscovered a love for running in those woods, explaining, "I start to recognize my body, and I run with light legs and stiff calves. I find the speed. I'm pleased when I've finished. This was fun." As he found, running offers a unique venue in which to experience transcendence. Of course, we don't all need to live and train alone in the woods to reveal it. This chapter is all about the power of running and the ways it can induce this extraordinary state of mind.

***

Balancing Work and Play

The types of optimal experiences I describe in this book arise in all sorts of environments. It's been touted as an important state to be able to access among a wide demographic, from rock climbers to musicians to surgeons. Multinational corporations and entire industries are implementing flow-based solutions to achieve increased performance, productivity, and happiness. As we begin to better understand the significance of this special state of consciousness, people are doing all manner of crazy things to "hack" flow—spinning around in human-sized gyroscopes and BASE jumping in wing suits.

But what if all you needed to do was go for a run?

We run for our health, to build fitness, to chase goals, and to make social connections. In some cultures, it's a way of life and a necessity of day-to-day survival. Indeed, anthropologist Allen Abramson touts running's "socio-cosmic" potential, elevating the many avenues through which the sport penetrates all class levels, working its way into the lifestyles of people across the globe.

As *Homo sapiens*, we've evolved to be some of the most accomplished running animals on the face of the Earth. It's part of who we are. It is our modern, sedentary existence for which we are not built. Indeed, thanks to the tectonically slow nature of evolution, our bodies remain primed for work and movement. When we run, we become who we were meant to be on a deep level.

Consider this: Even in our high-tech world of blazing fast supercomputers and mind-blowing inventions, experts struggle to design a robot that can compete with human runners. Scientists have figured out how to print next-generation spacecraft parts in three dimensions, grow synthetic embryos, cure some of the world's most feared diseases, and manufacture artificial hearts and self-driving cars. But we struggle to design sophisticated bipedal robots that can run efficiently. A highly complex process, just one step requires nerve signals to communicate with the rest of your body to direct it where to place your foot in relation to the slope of the ground, relative to the positioning of the rest of your body. Our innate running ability is lodged in our DNA—we as human beings just have to let our bodies run.

There's a reason legendary track star Steve Prefontaine likened running to a work of art. In 1977, David Shainberg, a renowned psychoanalyst, author, and runner, published a paper in the *Annals of the New York Academy of Sciences*, where he put it this way:

"When we run, we discover the sense in which nature is present in our bodies. Each morning there is a discovery of the texture and sinews of my muscles; the first steps of the run assert the presence of my connection to the rest of the matter of the universe. In one sense, as I run, it is clear that my body is mechanically organized and performs the functions of my run in a similar manner each day. I depend on the actualities of nature. The movements of running come along together, one after another once I go out there and run. I recognize my coordination each day and feel a kind of respect for the way it works together without my doing anything that puts it together."

Perhaps it is this deeply rooted link between humans and running that makes it such an apt venue by which to generate optimal experiences. In my research, I discovered that, while this state of consciousness can arise in all sorts of activities—from creative writing, to playing video games, to conversations between friends—the opportunity that running offers to balance mental and physical work with what experts call "play" make it distinctive.

From the world of education comes the term "hard fun," first coined by Seymour Papert, a South African-born mathematician and educator who was one of the pioneers of artificial intelligence. "Hard fun" encompasses the idea that we all enjoy a challenge, but only in activities in which we also find enjoyment and connection. It is thought that such activities have the potential to introduce the conditions necessary for optimal experiences to arise.

While hard-fun activities like writing a novel or playing a challenging computer game can certainly be venues in which optimal experiences come about, they are set apart from a physical sport like running—one that your entire being gets caught up in. Running provides a unique occasion for hard fun because it engages your mental and physical faculties, along with involving both fun and enjoyment. When you approach training with excitement to tackle a worthy challenge, but can also identify a sense of joy and adventure in the process, you set yourself up to experience that perfect running state. Let's take a look at these two components as they pertain to running: Work and play.

Work: Running as a Total Mind-Body Challenge

Through the warp and weft of life, we are constantly navigating the cognitive and emotional switchbacks of our own consciousness. Even if our psychic energy is well spent, we often feel at the mercy of outside forces. Genetics, politics, climate, the pull of gravity, the motion of the stars—there are so many things in life that are out of our control. It can be easy to feel that fate is preordained.

Even so, we have all had experiences where we had the sense we were in total control. These moments stick in our minds as profound. Interestingly, they don't generally occur in the comfort of your easy chair in your living room where you may have the perception of greater control. Rather, these moments that make life feel worthwhile occur when we are working hard, challenged, and stretched to our limits. This is a big reason that running makes such a supreme training ground for cultivating optimal experiences.

Physical skills are fundamental when it comes to most living beings. Think of a baby learning to crawl and walk. From an early age, physical competency is wired to enjoyment and satisfaction. For adults, running is an extension of that. Part of this can be explained by the fact that running requires effort. Even easy runs pose some level of challenge.

Indeed, research shows that the perceived challenge of an activity is a strong predictor of enjoyment. Studies even suggest that runners of all paces tend to prefer more difficult workouts over easy ones and that the satisfaction gained from that experience feeds intrinsic motivation. Regardless of your experience level as a runner or definition of what a "hard" workout is, running provides a constant state of work—the challenge to hit a pace, to reach the next mile marker without walking, to shatter a personal best, or qualify for a race. On some days, simply getting out the door for a run counts as a challenge overcome. Once you're up and running, there are always new opportunities to up the ante as your skillset improves and fitness builds.

What's more, each time you hit the road for a run, the activity also involves a test of your mental aptitude. Endurance running requires focus over a long period of time, an ability to visualize a performance in the midst of movement, and a creative willingness to engage a wellspring of toughness and positivity. In a race or hard workout, you're required to make split-second decisions about things like pace, nutritional intake, and tactical moves. New runners are faced with the challenge of learning to regulate physical discomfort and mental focus. While your mind will go into a less demanding headspace when you enter that perfect running state, leading up to it you're working to process, concentrate, and problem solve.

In psychology, Cognitive Evaluation Theory suggests that enjoyment of challenging activities is rooted in perceptions of competence—when we see ourselves as being skilled in an activity, we become motivated to repeatedly complete the task to work to improve further. Related studies have demonstrated that when people are engaging in an activity that they perceive as challenging in a skillful manner, they feel happier, stronger, more focused, and creative than during more passive leisure activities. It is in this space that those perfect runs arise.

As will be discussed further in Chapter 5, when the difficulty of the run and your skillset as an athlete match up, those perfect runs are more likely to materialize. On the one hand, you don't want the run to be so easy that you end up feeling bored and disengaged. At the same time, you also don't want it to be so challenging that you feel frustrated and give up. While a calculated amount of stress might help nurture optimal experiences, too much stress inhibits it. In fact, several researchers have noted that an overly competitive environment or mindset is a sure way to kill the chances of reaching this state of mind. That sweet spot, or channel of perfection, exists between boredom and frustration.

Play: Running as a Source of Fun

The other side of the equation in the realm of hard fun is the "fun" part. This is where the idea of "play" enters the picture. George Sheehan argued that to cultivate optimal experiences through running, one must view the activity as a strenuous form of play, claiming that a certain salvation could be found when you run for the pure joy of it, unconcerned by the outcome. He asserted that approaching running with an almost childlike affinity helps unify body and spirit, which is essential to satisfying training and finding meaning and happiness beyond the run.

Indeed, I've heard similar sentiments again and again in the hundreds of interviews I've conducted with runners over the years. In her memoir, Deena Kastor aptly describes this approach, writing about how she worked to get back to the mindset she harbored running as a youngster—envisioning herself as a puma crashing through the forest, a speeding car barreling down the road, a lioness at the start line, or a soldier on the front lines storming into battle. It was that mentality that allowed her to see running as a playful adventure.

The modern scholarly study of play can be traced back to Dutch historian and cultural theorist Johan Huizinga. In his 1938 book *Homo Ludens,* he argued for the central role of play in human culture, emphasizing that defining characteristics of play involve fun and enjoyment. His book describes play as an activity that is participated in for its own sake with no desire for material interest or profit, as well as one that is distinct from the constrictions of "real" life. Framing running as play offers the athlete a respite from daily life—an expanse of time where obligations and worries are suspended. In play, we break free of the ordinary and explore new potential and possibilities.

Markus Torgeby wrote about how transforming running into an activity that was less serious and more spontaneous and fun helped him rediscover a passion for the sport:

> *"I start to run across the marsh that angles downwards from the summit. I run fast on the downhill slope, increasing my speed until I lose control, fall over and slide on my stomach over the muddy grass and am soaked to the skin. I get up, carry on running and laugh aloud to myself. I'm feeling a bit crazy. Am I losing it? I don't give a damn. I lose control again and slip down into a muddy hollow. This is life. I'm completely consumed by nature."*

Desire Paths: An easy way to make running more playful is to go off-script on a run by taking what urban planners call "desire paths"— those made by people who trod off the beaten trail to forge their own way. They are often the paths of least resistance or those that take you on a more scenic route. There are many of these near my home in Minneapolis along rivers, lakes, and creeks. While I could stick to a perfectly groomed paved trail, I prefer to explore where the muddy footpaths through the woods take me.

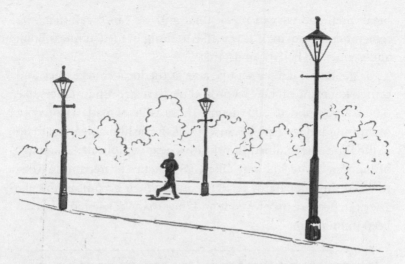

Balancing work and play in your running life can help you achieve perfection.

One of my favorite stories that demonstrates the importance of bringing a playful mindset to running comes from a piece I reported on back in 2010 about running in the 1960s in my home state of Minnesota. For the project, I was given a dusty old box of records, overflowing with brittle and yellow newspaper clippings and folders bound by rusty metal rings—most of the documents were a quarter of a century older than me at the time. While I was peripherally aware of the long line of great runners that hailed from my home state, I eagerly dug into the records and began interviewing the old timers around town.

Although running was viewed as a bizarre hobby by much of the general public at that time, these local runners, which included 1975 Boston Marathon runner-up Steve Hoag and Olympians Ron Daws and Van Nelson, ran purely for the love of the sport and they were forging new paths in the running history books along the way. One of the men I interviewed recalled thumbing through the Amateur Athletic Union (AAU) record books and picking out new American records they thought they could set. "We can break that, and we can break that, and we can break that," he remembered thinking. "It was like looking in the Guinness Book and saying, 'oh hell, I can do that!'"

For the fun of it, they set up races at the local college track and started knocking off new records, often at lesser-run distances like 6,000, 8,000, and 30,000 meters. These athletes made a game out of running and it wasn't because it was the fashionable thing to do at the time. They trained in primitive gear without the advantage of modern-day technology, like GPS watches or treadmills. They received little fanfare or recognition for their accomplishments. They ran because they loved it and they made concerted efforts to keep training fun.

Making Running Fun Again: How can you transform your running routine from a solely competitive endeavor or humdrum exercise regimen into something more playful and appealing? Approaching runs with a sense of energy, enthusiasm, and spontaneity is imperative. Making simple adjustments to your running routine can spark a spirit of play that injects new life into your workouts. If your runs are feeling more like work than play, try one of the following:

- Run a new route
- Sign up to race a new distance
- Take part in a themed race
- Recruit a new running partner
- Join a running group
- Ditch your watch for a week and run by feel

A hallmark of play is full absorption in a task. I think of my daughter when she's immersed in imaginative play with her toy horses and trucks. Say her name and she won't respond. Try to convince her to wrap up the activity and she'll resist. Children have a unique ability to slip into their own make-believe worlds. As adults, we often lose that playful mindset, missing out on these opportunities to lose ourselves in enjoyable activities. To be sure, experts suggest that the deep involvement that comes along with play can help an individual reach flow.

Absorption and the perfect running state can't be forced or manufactured. Think of a hard workout where things aren't coming together and you feel like you're pushing through sheer force of will. These are the moments that require grit to keep plodding forward. There's no ease or finesse in movement, just the feeling of muscling through. Conversely, when you are fully involved in a run, everything clicks and energy courses through your body, naturally propelling you forward. Some days this will inexplicably arise and other days it won't.

Torgeby writes this of his running philosophy:

"For many, running becomes a matter of consumption, a matter that has to be accounted for and be superseded. Just another achievement in a life that is all about achieving things on every level. I believe that that sort of thinking is mistaken. Freedom in movement disappears if it is reduced to something comparative. It becomes bureaucracy, running in ordered rows along a fixed, predetermined path. Running is the movement of a free human being. It doesn't demand any special premises or machines. You only need to put on your shoes and get going. Let the blood circulate. Then everything becomes much clearer."

After four years spent living and running in the woods, Torgeby emerged a different man. Twenty years hence, he lives with his wife and two children in a cottage in the mountain pastures not far from his former base camp in the woods. The impact of discovering a more playful approach to running continues to impact his life well beyond the miles. Indeed, now a lecturer and author recognized as a guru of long-distance and trail running, he welcomes visitors for several days to his home to discuss these themes. He writes of these visitors: "Together we live the simple life—making fires, preparing food outside and washing ourselves in the sauna after several hours of running. Living the life that helped me to make my head connect with my body—a life that can benefit everyone. A few days without stress, where running becomes a way of opening up your heart." Upon being asked what makes life worth living, he adds, "I know only that the forest and running happened to help me find my way."

When you approach running with a playful mindset and pair that with adequate challenge, you structure running to be an exercise in hard fun. This provides a unique opportunity for optimal experiences to arise, but even so, perfection isn't guaranteed. The next four chapters will look at the main factors that contribute to perfection in running: Presence, purpose, planning, and process.

Practices in Perfection

- Running is part of who we are on an evolutionary level.
- The sport offers a unique opportunity for optimal experiences because it balances mental and physical work with play.
- The challenge of a run must be well matched to the skill of the runner to elicit perfect running experiences.
- When running is viewed as a playful adventure, it separates it from "real" life and transforms it into a prime opportunity for perfect running experiences to materialize.

Chapter 3
PRESENCE

*"I just thought about the next moment. I don't wake up
and think about running 3o–35 miles, I just get started.
If you can get past those mental barriers, you can
accomplish amazing things."*

A MONTH BEFORE the Tour de France riders arrived to take
on the Pyrenees, Zoë Romano made her way up a craggy green
mountainside on foot. Hamstrings and calves screaming, she
moved over the cold asphalt under an overcast sky. Soon this road
would be a spectacle—packed with colorful fans and spandex-
clad riders—all broadcast to a global audience. But today, it was
just Romano and the road.

In 2013, the then 26-year-old decided she wanted to be the first
person to run the entire 2,000-mile (3,220-km) Tour de France
course. To do this, she started before the riders and calculated
she'd have to log the 21 stages at an average nine-minute-mile
pace over nine weeks. That meant running 30 miles (48 km) a
day and taking on more than 100,000 feet (30,000 meters) of
elevation change.

A teacher based in Richmond, Virginia, Romano was no stranger
to feats of endurance. In 2011, she became the first woman to
run 3,000 miles (4,830 km) across the U.S. from Huntington
Beach, California, to Charleston, South Carolina, pushing all her

belongings in a running stroller as she raised money for charity. In search of a new challenge and a fresh method of funding for a cause she cared about, running the Tour de France came up as a possibility.

I caught up with her six weeks into her Tour journey for a story I was working on and she told me this: "If you want to do something no one else has done before, you have to put yourself out there. This was a really personal mission of mine, and it was out in public. Being willing to say that I was intimidated and didn't know if I could do it helped me make the leap in the first place."

The first major test in the Pyrenees was served up courtesy of Col de Pailhères. It involved nearly 10 miles (16 km) of climbing at an average 8.2 percent grade. To put that into perspective, most gym treadmills max out at around 10 percent grade. Romano began the intimidating climb, not by focusing on the summit, but rather on the next subsequent step and breath. Only then would she make the necessary progress without being overwhelmed by the entirety of the task. "I just thought about the next moment. I don't wake up and think about running 30–35 miles, I just get started," she told me. "If you can get past those mental barriers, you can accomplish amazing things."

As she made her way up the mountain, the grade and length of the climb became a relentless and punishing task. Her legs ached and her mind fought to stay focused on putting one foot in front of the other. With each passing mile, though, that heaviness made way for a sense of levity. "It began to feel maybe not easy, but comfortable. I felt prepared and trained and the miles were going by more quickly than usual," she recalled to me a few years later. "It's a weird feeling, being totally in the experience, knowing you're physically in pain, but not being attached to that pain. When I entered those moments of true flow, it felt like this unending dance where I wasn't hyperaware of everything. I was just in the run."

She said that she often repeated a mantra once uttered by her mother: "This is what we are doing now." Instead of fighting against or denying the discomfort and boredom associated with the challenge, she put her energy toward mentally committing to the process and making headway up the mountain.

The air was thin up at the top of the high mountain pass, but Romano's body, which was stiff and tired that morning when she awoke, somehow cruised effortlessly as she reached the 6,500-foot (1,980-km) summit. Revealing a stunning panorama of the Pyrenees, she felt like she could run for days, which is exactly what she would do, except for stops for food and rest.

"The Pyrenees were a daunting, but motivational challenge. There's nothing like running across a mountain range," she said. "I felt incredible at the top of every mountain. Every time I paused to think about the fact that I could get to the tops of these mountains day after day by my own two feet. There's this, 'I can't believe I just did that' feeling. I know that incomparable feeling I

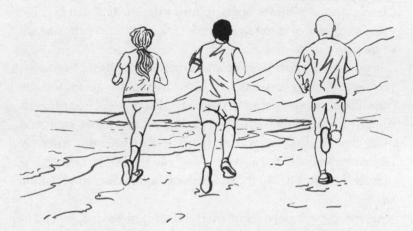

A mindful approach to running can make way for reaching an optimal headspace.

got when I reached the top continued to drive many of my steps in the mountains in France."

Romano's successful Tour de France run offers a prescient example of how, no matter the challenge, remaining present can make way for perfect running experiences. This chapter will delve into why a mindful approach to your training is so important, along with presenting actionable steps to bring greater presence to your running practice.

* * *

Building a Mindful Foundation

At its core, mindfulness is about focusing your attention on the present moment without judgment. A concept largely introduced to Western audiences back in the 1980s by Dr. Jon Kabat-Zinn of the University of Massachusetts Medical School, it's been taught in schools, hospitals, and boardrooms, all with an aim to reduce the ailments and inefficiencies associated with a wandering, chaotic, and sometimes undisciplined mind. It has also become increasingly relied upon to improve experience and performance in sports.

Renowned Danish thinker and existential philosopher Søren Kierkegaard suggested that our general impulse to escape the present through perpetual activity and distraction is our biggest source of unhappiness. To be sure, studies show that we spend more than half of our waking hours lost in thought, endlessly worrying and obsessing about the past and future. We rarely allow ourselves to "just be" in the moment or, in this case, run the mile we are in.

Recent research out of Harvard University shows that we tend to be happiest when we are fully absorbed in a task in the moment.

Mindfulness builds that muscle of attention by calling you to focus on the present moment and any time you notice your mind has wandered, to redirect it back to the moment. This allows you to recognize what's occurring in the present and respond in the most productive way possible. It trains the mind to eschew extraneous distractions and unproductive thinking and center attention on the act of running.

Mindfulness also helps build intrinsic motivation, resilience, optimism, gratitude, and a process-focused attitude. Having the wherewithal to persist, even on the far-from-flowy days when you're slogging more than soaring, can help lead to important breakthroughs in your training that reveal those transcendent moments. When I spoke with Michael Gervais, a high-performance psychologist known for his work with the NFL's Seattle Seahawks and Austrian skydiver Felix Baumgartner, he likened it to rowing a raft down a river. If you notice rapids up ahead and you want to avoid them because they might slow you down or cause you to tip, it is mindful awareness that can help you steer clear of the turbulence.

Similarly, Adrienne Taren, a neuroscientist and mindfulness researcher at the University of Pittsburgh, once told me this: "Mindfulness gives you a flashlight and you have control over where you point that flashlight. You can direct your attention or flashlight away from panicky or ruminative thoughts and emotional responses and shine it somewhere more productive. It's not that those thoughts aren't there, you just learn to peacefully coexist by not shining the light on them."

Indeed, your life experiences are largely shaped by how you allocate your attention. Very different realities emerge depending on whether the direction of your attention is intentional and focused or more scattered and random. Consider the following three possible mindsets a runner might have on race day. Which do you think would most likely lead to an optimal running experience and performance?

1. The obsessive runner: This athlete constantly worries about things like that soreness in her knee, if she trained hard enough, the water stops on the course, and whether her goals will be perfectly met.

2. The distracted runner: This athlete is constantly thinking about anything other than the race at hand. He's making a grocery list, thinking about the paperwork piling up on his desk back at the office, and worrying about a fight he had with a friend last week.

3. The mindful runner: This athlete is paying attention to the in-and-out of her breath and her foot strike. She notices the angle of the sun and the impressive landscape around her. She makes decisions about pace with intention and precision. When her mind does wander, she quickly notices and returns her focus to the present moment.

Moment-to-moment awareness always precedes perfect running experiences. Without it, a positive attitude, high motivation, and lofty goals may get you out the door, but won't elevate you to that next-level headspace. Gervais told me this: "Mindfulness is a defining feature of elite athletes. So if you want to get better, best practices would suggest, do what the best do. Research shows that those who practice mindfulness have an increased frequency of flow states—the most optimal state a human can be in."

The neuroscientist who was introduced in Chapter 1, Leslie Sherlin, put it to me this way:

"It can be hard for athletes because so much of sport is about self-evaluation—it can be challenging to get out of your head and away from thinking, 'how's my time?',

'what's my pace?' and just be in the moment experiencing it. Mindfulness is really a core component of flow state. Even from the early writings of Csikszentmihalyi when he was starting to describe flow states and developing a model of the prerequisites to achieving the flow state, all of them included the concept of experiencing the moment as it was happening and in a nonjudgmental way. Just by definition, if you aren't being mindful, you won't experience flow."

Whether or not you're concerned about performance, mindfulness is key to cultivating a positive running experience. A mentality of presence can pave the way for perfection when you're going out for a relaxed run around your neighborhood or racing at the top level of the sport.

Exercise 3.1: How to Practice Mindfulness
Choosing an anchor for your attention can be a great first step in your mindfulness practice. Set aside a few moments of a run to complete a basic meditation. Select either your in-and-out breath or your footfall as your anchor to the present moment. For those few minutes, train your attention on that anchor. Examine the intricacies of your breath or the sensation of your feet hitting the ground. Every time you notice your mind has wandered to something other than focusing on your anchor, gently bring your attention back to your breathing or footfall. You will likely find your mind will become distracted over and over again, but with time and practice, your attention will remain more readily focused on your anchor without as much effort. This, in a nutshell, is what mindfulness is all about.

----

* * *

How Mindfulness Promotes Perfection

Romano chose to run the final 90 miles (145 km) of the Tour de France course all in one go—finishing her journey with an almost 24-hour run straight through. When I spoke to her soon after her finish, she told me, "This just feels surreal because there were so many times I had doubts and felt uncertain. There were times when I could hardly imagine being able to finish on time and in one piece. It feels impossible that it has actually happened."

While the hardest, most gut-wrenching moments of her 2,000-mile run were memorable, those brushes with perfection—and the present-moment awareness that facilitated them—kept her going day in and day out. Those are also the snapshots that linger in her mind years later, continuing to give shape and meaning to her life. More recently, she told me this:

> *"Being open to the moment-to-moment experience in France was part of the fun—I didn't know I was going to run into a wild boar out there on the first week, or meet all these amazing people along the way, or run through fields of lavender. Every day there were so many bizarre and beautiful experiences that had nothing to do with running. Long term, that journey taught me that while you might know you're going to get from point A to point B, you don't know what's going to happen in between and that's okay."*

While, by her nature, Romano is motivated by big goals, the many singular moments along that Tour de France route were what eventually added up to her successful completion of it. "Having a big picture goal, the idea of doing something no one had ever done and I didn't know if I could do, was very motivating," she explained. "But every day I woke up and just focused on the small things and what I needed to do in that moment and on that day."

As Romano's experience illustrates, rather than wasting energy trying to suppress or eliminate distracting thoughts and emotions, mindfulness trains the brain to take note and move on to more important things in the moment. Research has shown that as little as six weeks of mindfulness training increases flow scores, and the likelihood an athlete will encounter optimal experiences, by offering an enhanced ability to focus on performance over distractions, and better accept the inherent ups and downs that accompany just about any activity. To be sure, there are a number of specific ways that mindfulness primes a runner to experience more perfect running:

Mindfulness breeds focus and self-discipline

As we've learned, supreme focus is a trademark of the perfect running state. In a review of the current literature on flow and sport, experts identified a number of common findings. Chief among them was the ability to sustain attention during a task. When your mind is wandering, you are anything but focused, your body falls out of sync, and the quality of the running experience suffers. Mindfulness opens up the opportunity for perfect running experiences by promoting prolonged concentration. Research demonstrates that just five days of 20 minutes a day of mindfulness meditation has the potential to significantly fortify your ability to focus.

What's more, when examining the personality traits that make a person more likely to encounter optimal experiences, Swedish researchers found that conscientiousness rose to the top. When you have an enhanced ability to remain focused on the task of running, you're more apt to stick to your training plan and less likely to get derailed by distractions and impulsivities. The Mayo Clinic's Michael Joyner, one of the world's top experts on the physiology of human endurance, put it to me this way:

"I've found flow is an important part of achieving optimal performance in anything I do—I use some of the same techniques I use in training when writing grants and doing clinical procedures. In all cases, it involves intense and focused effort to achieve a task. It requires you to be completely in the moment, but you also lose track of time—you look up and an hour or two has passed without you realizing it."

Exercise 3.2: Mindful Shoe Tying

Establishing a mindful focus takes practice, so why not start with something easy? The next time you go to put on your running shoes for a workout, pause for a moment and reflect. Pay attention to how the lace feels in your hand. Feel the upper of the shoe tightening around your foot. Watch as you tie the knot. Notice how it feels once it's tied. This sounds ridiculously simple, but it can have a profound impact when it comes to setting the stage for a more present-focused run.

Mindfulness boosts emotional intelligence

Emotional intelligence has to do with your ability to identify, manage, and respond to your emotions and the emotions of others. A major tenet of mindfulness is the practice of observing thoughts, but then being able to redirect to the present moment. It trains you to respond rather than react to things, putting higher order thought in the driver's seat rather than the lizard brain, which is compelled by the fight-flight-freeze response. This in turn helps to buffer the stress response and boost higher reasoning to

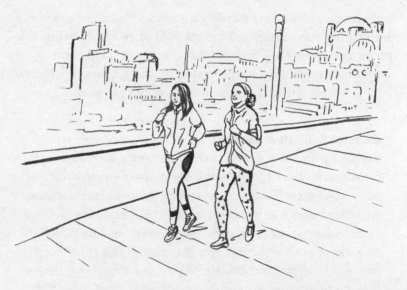

Mindful running helps sow the seeds of perfection.

keep you on track toward your goals. The sense of equanimity that is sowed is integral to emotional intelligence.

Emotional intelligence has been shown to be a significant predictor of optimal experiences. Researchers have identified three main ways that mindfulness builds emotional intelligence: (1) It helps you hone the ability to identify and understand your emotions, (2) It boosts your awareness and recognition of the emotions of those around you, and (3) It improves your ability to control your emotions. These are all advantages in performance situations where emotions can run high. In fact, one study on emotional intelligence that surveyed runners before a half marathon discovered that scores predicted finishing times more accurately than training history.

The thought is that when you rank highly in emotional intelligence, you're better at dealing with the myriad of emotions you might face during a run or race. Just because you had a slow mile doesn't mean you should get mad and quit. So you had a leg cramp? Stay steady, walk it off, and start again. Being able to effectively identify and regulate emotions helps you avoid becoming consumed by rumination and negativity in order to problem solve and keep pushing when things get hard.

Exercise 3.3: Affect Labeling

We often get stuck in a cycle of either becoming overwhelmed by our emotions or trying to ignore or suppress them. Mindfulness helps you become aware of these feelings in real time through a process referred to as "affect labeling." Set aside five minutes to sit in silence with your eyes closed. Take the first minute to slow down your breathing and get comfortable. Then begin to pay attention to the content of your thinking. Every time a thought or emotion crosses your landscape of consciousness, label it with a word that describes the emotion attached to it, and then let it float along through your mind without focusing on it. For instance, say you begin to ruminate about a negative conversation you had with your boss last week—label it "anger," and go back to focusing on an anchor in the present moment. Next, maybe you notice how much your shoulders ache from the constant stress you've been experiencing. Label it "tension." Continue the exercise for another several minutes. Recognizing and identifying emotions has a way of eliminating their power.

Mindfulness emphasizes intrinsic motivation

While intrinsic motivation will be covered in more depth in Chapter 4, it's worth mentioning in relation to mindfulness. Csikszentmihalyi described flow as "autotelic," which means that the experience is the reward in and of itself. Indeed, runners who are driven by intrinsic motivation are more likely to encounter perfect running experiences. These types of runners are engaged in training, motivated by the sheer love of the sport, and are not overly concerned with achievements and accolades.

French researchers discovered that mindfulness can increase an athlete's intrinsic motivation to train and compete. This is probably in large part due to the fact that instead of getting lost in thought, it trains you to tune in to the moment-to-moment joys of running. The gorgeous scenery, the happy exhaustion that accompanies a well-executed workout, or the simple freedom of movement all constitute as intrinsically motivating reasons to run—and ones that can lead to that perfect running experience.

Exercise 3.4: Triumphs and Tweaks

Every run and race has its ups and downs. Unfortunately, we often end up obsessing about the lower points. Negativity has a way of sapping purpose and intrinsic motivation from your running practice. Next time you finish a workout, sit down for a couple of minutes and list three things you think you did well and three things you might tweak during the next workout. This list acknowledges the fact that you're constantly building and it's okay to identify weaknesses, but it also helps to emphasize the things that you're doing well to keep you coming back for more.

Mindfulness bolsters resilience and stress tolerance

One major impediment to achieving that perfect running state is stress. This was a prominent theme among the runners I surveyed. Among the things that could prevent flow, they reported: "Pressure to perform," "worrying about numbers," "feeling pressed for time and distracted," "unreasonable expectations and a busy mind," and "feeling rushed, unprepared, or distracted." When you're stressed, your body releases cortisol, which in turn increases heart rate and adrenaline levels, interfering with physical performance and clear thinking. Stress takes you out of the moment and bogs you down in worries and anxieties, making perfect running experiences all but out of reach.

Mindfulness helps athletes view anxious thoughts with a mind of acceptance, which has been shown to improve performance. The alternative approach is to simply expend energy trying to ignore or resist the stressful thoughts, inevitably giving them greater power. Research involving NCAA athletes found that a brief mindfulness intervention lowered stress levels. Alternatively, another study found that an open and receptive attitude allowed athletes to cope more adeptly with the ups and downs of training.

Exercise 3.5: Tension Inventory

Set aside ten minutes of your day to sit in a chair with a straight back and your hands resting gently in your lap. Close your eyes and begin to slowly scan from your head down to your toes. Bring awareness to tightness and discomfort in each region of the body. If you notice tension, pause for a moment and see if simply focusing on it and examining it offers release. With practice, this exercise can help you not only relieve stress, but also build better body awareness.

Mindfulness builds gratitude

Counteracting our culture's emphasis on multitasking and constant activity, mindfulness trains your brain to embrace something called "soft fascination," which will be discussed further in Chapter 8. It is in those moments of mindfully cultivated soft fascination that awe, wonder, and gratitude are built. You're more likely to notice the sun warming your face and feel grateful for the ability to run. These joy-inducing moments of gratitude put you firmly in the moment on a run, setting the stage for the perfect running experience.

According to scientists, the feeling of awe has a unique link to well-being. Awe—your response to something vast that changes your frame of reference—creates a sense of "self-diminishment," which basically means that it offers you a glimpse of yourself as part of something larger. Researchers have demonstrated that this feeling of connection even has the ability to boost immune system health and bolster overall well-being.

Exercise 3.6: Gratitude Journal

As you work to harness greater mindfulness in running and life, you'll naturally begin to notice things for which you are grateful. Keeping an ongoing list has been shown to increase happiness and optimism. To do this, designate a journal or notebook and jot down three things you are grateful for each day. This could be as simple as your morning cup of hot coffee or a great run with a friend. Even the seemingly small moments of happiness in your day are worth noting. With some practice, you'll likely find yourself seeking out and recognizing examples of gratitude in order to write them down later.

Mindfulness reduces self-judgment

Self-judgment and its close cousins, self-consciousness and self-criticism, can all eliminate the chances of accessing a perfect run. Not only do they cause you to underestimate your capabilities, they also signal a lack of focus. Obsessing about how you look to other people or getting down on yourself for a lackluster mile simply serve as distractions.

Interestingly, new research shows that mindful individuals naturally deactivate a region of the brain that is responsible for self-referential processes, which are often associated with rumination and anxiety. Mindfulness can help you remain focused on what is directly in front of you in the present moment, rather than jumping down the rabbit hole of obsessive thoughts and anxieties, thereby increasing the likelihood of discovering those perfect runs.

Exercise 3.7: Mindful Breathing

Mindful breathing exercises can be a great way to slow down self-referential thought processes and refocus on the present moment. Set aside at least five minutes in a quiet place and try one of these exercises:

- Matching breath: Start by inhaling through your nose as you count in your head 1-2-3-4. Then exhale 1-2-3-4. As you become more relaxed, see if you can slow your breathing rate down and count to 5 or 6.
- Belly breathing: Sitting with a straight back and good posture, take a deep breath. Feel your belly inflate as you focus on your abdomen before allowing the breath to fill your chest. Then exhale, relaxing your belly and continuing for several minutes.
- Breath counting: Focus on breathing in deeply, filling your lungs completely. Pause and then slowly expel all of the air out of your lungs as you exhale. That is one round. Continue to count each round up to 20.

Mindfulness cultivates a process-focused attitude

There's plenty of academic and anecdotal evidence to support the fact that athletes tend to experience flow and perform at their best when they are focused on process rather than outcome.

Psychologist and author of *Mindset: The New Psychology of Success*, Carol Dweck references the "growth mindset," which is all about embracing the ups and downs of the process with the knowledge that it is all valuable to growth. On the flip side, a "fixed mindset" is characterized by the belief that your abilities are set in stone. As you might expect, the growth mindset is more conducive to motivation. What's more, research shows that when athletes are overly concerned about their end goal, they often have their worst performances.

Of course, runners of all experience levels and ambitions find themselves clinging to certain goals and becoming obsessed with outcomes at one point or another. Mindfulness helps you identify these well-worn patterns of thought in order to shift mindset and remain on a path of continuous growth.

Exercise 3.8: Running Reflection

At the beginning of each of your runs this week, spend the first few minutes reflecting on what part that specific workout plays in the larger scheme of things. For instance, the function of your long run is to build endurance, your weight-training sessions will build strength, your track workouts will build speed, and your rest day will allow for important physiological adaptations to take hold. Understanding the role of each aspect of training can help create a foundation of respect for the process. When you understand why you are doing what you're doing on a daily basis and view training as a long game, you're less likely to get derailed by setbacks.

Mindfulness opens you to new experiences

People who rank high in something psychologists call "openness," defined as the intellectual curiosity and motivation to explore inner and outer experiences, tend to search out new experiences more readily. Mindfulness is key to cultivating openness because it fosters an attitude of nonjudgmental awareness, which is largely about taking in the spectrum of life experiences with a mind of acceptance.

Research has linked openness to all sorts of constructs that are related to optimal experiences. For example, studies demonstrate that people open to new and unusual experiences are more susceptible to becoming absorbed in flow-inducing tasks. Openness is also correlated with positive affect and quality of life, which similarly helps set the stage for perfect running. Since it can be a wholly elevated and even somewhat strange experience, being open to unexpected perfection on a run is essential.

Exercise 3.9: Open Awareness Meditation

On your next run, devote the first 5–10 minutes to noticing your surroundings. Utilize your five senses as you take in the full landscape of what's around you.

- What do you hear? Are there horns honking? An airplane overhead? Just the sound of the soft breeze?
- What do you smell? Are there restaurants or fast-food joints nearby that give off a certain aroma? What about the scents of nature—flowers blooming or rotting leaves?
- What do you taste? Do you sometimes get a metallic tang in your mouth when you run? Does your mouth feel dry?
- What do you feel? Is rain falling and soaking through your running clothes? Is the wind blowing your hood back? Is the ground underfoot soft or hard?
- What do you see? What colors, shapes, and textures are around you? Are there people, houses, or cars zipping by? Is there much in the way of nature to observe?

---

* * *

The Steps to Becoming a More Mindful Runner

In my first book, *Mindful Running*, I lay out in detail a mindful running process that I call "Focus, Fathom, Flow," which describes the cycle of first mindfully tuning in to a run, then pondering if any adjustments need to be made, and finally, if all goes well, you enter the flow state. I repeat the first two actionable steps in the upcoming pages.

You've probably heard the axiom "neurons that fire together wire together." It's an abridged description of Canadian psychologist Donald Hebb's theory that when neurons in the brain fire at the same time, they become associated with one another. Over time and repetition, the brain adapts to these repeated patterns of firing, thereby developing a new skill. As the skill is practiced, pathways continue to strengthen and actions and responses become second nature. In the same way that your brain creates and runs a neuro-circuit every time it executes a line of thinking, emotion, or activity, so too will it fire up a network of neurons when you experience a perfect run. Even on the runs when you don't enter deep flow, you can lay the groundwork for perfect running to become more accessible.

It stands to reason that the more often you enter that perfect running state, the easier it becomes to reach. Indeed, 2004 Olympic silver medalist and winner of the 2009 New York City Marathon and 2014 Boston Marathon, Meb Keflezighi, told me this: "Achieving flow doesn't happen with the snap of a finger. As an athlete I get there through movement. After a period of time, my mind starts to tune out distractions and I slip into that elevated state. Today, with so many years of experience, I can even get there on regular training runs."

By training your mind to cycle through the appropriate steps to reach a more mindful state, you create the conditions for perfect runs to arise. Here are the basics:

Step 1: Focus

The focus phase of a run should come toward the beginning. It's all about dialing in to the present moment as you run and becoming more attuned to your body, your mind, and the world around you. I like to describe this as "dropping in" to the presence of a run and fully immersing yourself in the act of movement.

As has been mentioned, focus is a theme that comes up repeatedly in the literature investigating optimal experiences. Indeed, in systematic reviews of this state, the ability to direct attention for prolonged periods of time is identified as one of the most important triggers. As Michael Gervais told me, "We want to be able to have the volitional control to guide our mind and body in the most effective way."

During this initial step, work to teach your mind to fully focus on certain aspects of the run, setting aside worries about the past or future, to-do lists, and planning. I suggest running through these three scanning exercises as you settle in to your run to bring greater focus to the activity. In total, these scans only take a few minutes to complete. If you become distracted, simply take note that your mind has wandered and return your focus to the exercise again and again.

Environmental scan

- What do you hear? Begin by noticing any sounds. If you're in the city, you may first hear the distant roar of an airplane overhead or the flow of traffic from a nearby highway. On a trail, singing birds or the howling wind might be more prominent. One of my favorite sounds I encounter on runs in Minnesota comes from ice melting on the lakes in the spring. Haunting reverberations echo across the frozen surface as the ice thaws and shifts. There will also be the sounds of your footsteps and respiration. Remember, don't impose expectations on how your foot strike or breathing should sound, just listen.

- What do you smell? Next, shift your attention to your sense of smell. It could be fresh-baked bread from a bakery, like the one in my neighborhood, or even a fast-food joint along your route. Depending on the time of year, certain scents from nature will be more obvious. I always love taking in the smell of blooming lilacs in the spring and the drying leaves in the fall.

- What do you taste? Observe any discernible flavors. This is easy if you're fueling with nutritionals or sports drinks, but those aren't the only tastes you'll necessarily come across. For instance, in the winter I've perceived a distinct brininess to the air after city crews spread salt on icy roads. Other times those tastes come from within. That metallic tang you get during an intense workout is thought to be from the red blood cells that accumulate in the lungs during hard efforts.

- What do you feel? Bring your focus to your sense of touch next. Perhaps you just wiped sweat from your brow and came away with a gritty residue. Or maybe you stopped at a drinking fountain to splash cold water on your face and tie your shoe. You'll also feel your feet as they make contact with the ground.

- What do you see? Take in the scenery. Notice the colors, shapes, and textures of the landscape. Check out the terrain underfoot. Focus on other runners or cyclists on the trail as they pass in the opposite direction. I always make sure to spend a few moments watching my dog, Welly, trotting a few feet ahead of me, her tail wagging and ears flopping with each bound. It's hard not to appreciate the moment when I watch her run.

Body scan

- Start at the top of your head. Bring your awareness to your scalp, forehead, eyes, and face. Are you holding any tension in your jaw or furrowing your brow? See if you can let it soften.
- Move down to your neck and shoulders. Are you tight, relaxed, or somewhere in between?
- Take note of your breath and the air filling your lungs. Are you inhaling and exhaling through both your nose and mouth? Is the air warm or cold?
- How do your arms, hands, and fingers feel? What is your arm carriage like? Are you using your arms to power forward?
- Next, scan down your spine. How is your posture? Are you hunching forward or slightly arching your back?
- Move on to your core, including your lower back, abdominals, and hips. Do you feel your hips rotating excessively or mostly driving forward? Are your abs engaged as you stride?
- Travel down your legs, taking stock of your quads, hamstrings, knees, shins, and calves. Are there any twinges of pain or discomfort? Do your legs feel fresh or tired?
- Finally, finish by observing your feet. Are you striking the ground with your heel, midfoot, or forefoot? Can you feel them roll inward as you make contact with the ground?

Mind scan

- Start by noticing and acknowledging the top three thoughts running through your mind.
- Take stock of the speed of your thoughts. Is your mind racing, are you feeling more lethargic, or are you somewhere in between?
- Identify whether you're attaching emotions to the thoughts. Are you worrying about work or stressing about what you have to do after the run?

- What is the storyline you're following? Are the thoughts you're having being fed by a certain identity you've created for yourself?
- Notice whether stress in your everyday life is shaping your attitude toward your run. Are the anxieties stemming from other venues causing you to feel bored, hurried, tired, or uncomfortable?
- Remember, being mindful is all about noticing the thoughts without judgment. Identify each thought as it pops into your head and let it move along without obsessing over it, trying to push it away, or clinging to it.

Step 2: Fathom

One of the keys of mindfulness training is not only training yourself to notice how things are in the present moment, but also having the wisdom to respond appropriately. For instance, via your mental scan, you may have noticed that you were cycling a long list of negative thoughts about yourself, rather than focusing on the run. Not only is negative self-talk a proven flow-killer, it can also be a self-fulfilling prophesy. In this step, you might decide to acknowledge this line of thinking and then redirect to the in-the-moment experience of the run. You could choose to focus on the in-and-out of your breath or the left-right-left of your feet.

Similarly, if during the body scan you noticed that your calves were screaming as you ran up a hill, this phase calls you to reflect on whether those sensations are the discomfort associated with hard running or an oncoming injury. If you conclude the former in this case, work to accept the inherent suffering that comes along with running and again redirect your attention to the in-the-moment experience. However, if you decide that your ailing calves are part of a larger pattern of pain and might signal an injury, the best course of action is likely to cut the run short.

The fathom phase can come in especially handy during races. For example, if you notice that your shoulders are tight, thereby throwing off your gait, you might choose to shake out your arms and relax your posture. Or if you notice your mouth is dry or you're feeling low on energy, you may decide to take in calories and hydration sooner than you originally planned. Reflecting on whatever is happening in the moment allows you to make adjustments on the fly. "With greater awareness, we become better attuned to adjusting more quickly to the internal and external demands and pressures of performance," Gervais explained to me.

Running is essentially an exercise in problem-solving. The ability to diagnose and fix whatever isn't going right in the moment can turn a terrible run into at least an okay run and maybe even a perfect one. If you face some sort of challenge—a bad mile, a leg cramp, stomach issues—it's about working to see if you can address and adjust, rather than continuing down a destructive path or throwing in the towel.

Laurence Gonzales, a journalist and author of *Deep Survival*, explains that to do this we rely on a system of "emotional bookmarks." If we can train ourselves to respond to certain types of stimuli in specific ways, we create a bookmark for that action. When you figure out how to mindfully deal with discomfort in a race instead of backing off at the first sign of fatigue, you generate a bookmark for that situation and response. This is all about training the mind to direct the body to do what you want it to do in the heat of the moment without too much cognitive engagement or debate. When you practice this in training, you strengthen the neural pathways for dealing with the myriad of issues that can come up during a run or race, thereby making the most productive response your go-to bookmark.

The power of mindfulness can be put to work before you even take that first step toward a perfect run. In Chapter 4 we'll look at how this mindset can help you discover greater purpose and authenticity in your approach to running.

Practices in Perfection

- A mindful approach to training is foundational to cultivating the right conditions for perfect running experiences to arise.
- Mindfulness involves harnessing a nonjudgmental focus on the present moment. When you notice your mind has wandered, it simply calls you to redirect to what's in front of you.
- Mindfulness facilitates perfect running experiences via increased focus, and self-discipline, superior emotional intelligence, greater intrinsic motivation, increased resilience to stress, gratitude, confidence, a process-focused attitude, and an enhanced openness to new experiences.
- To employ the first two steps of the mindful running process, Focus and Fathom, you must first tune in to the present moment of a run and then ponder if any adjustments need to be made.

Chapter 4
PURPOSE

"No matter the conditions, when I'm in flow, I'm totally focused on my footwork and using all my senses. I get into a rhythm as I'm listening to my feet and breathing. I'm not thinking about anything in particular, just hearing and feeling."

AS 52-YEAR-OLD PROFESSIONAL ultra-distance runner Diane Van Deren made her way down the thin, serpentine road known as North Carolina Highway 12 on May 30, 2012, she steeled herself against the high winds of Tropical Storm Beryl. The salty waters and piling waves of the Atlantic Ocean breached the asphalt strip as Van Deren and her running guide tethered themselves to one another with pack straps to avoid getting blown into the salt marsh on either side of the road.

As the region was shredded by 40-mile-per-hour (64kph) winds and more than a half-foot (15cm) of rain, lightning cracked and thunder made the ground beneath their feet shudder like a freight train. Akin to running face-first into an unmanned fire hose, the mix of ocean water, marshy debris, and beach sand stung every inch of their bodies. In pursuit of the 1 p.m. Cedar Island Ferry across Pamlico Sound to Ocracoke Island, they knew they had to keep moving if they wanted to catch their ride.

Van Deren entered a distinct state of consciousness as they navigated that stretch of land. "No matter what, I tried to stay steady and not let anything rock my boat. I didn't waste energy on feeling frustrated, tired, or mad about the conditions," she told me years later. "When you're running through a hurricane, you have a heightened sense of awareness. It's like riding a horse, galloping hard and then all of a sudden turning on to a different trail and pulling back on the reins. That's how you stay in the flow."

With only moments to spare, they reached the ferry. "You must have just come through those tornadoes back there!" shouted the ferry operator over the howling winds as they boarded. Van Deren smiled as she grabbed a towel and sat down to enjoy the ride. She had just completed a 36-mile (58-km) day on foot, day 10 of a three-week-long, 1,175-mile (1,891-km) journey across the entire state of North Carolina, known as the Mountains-to-Sea Trail.

Like much of the press on Van Deren, a story I penned about her for The Atlantic back in 2014 focused on the epilepsy diagnosis she received more than 30 years ago, which led to brain surgery— a lobectomy to remove a plum-sized portion of her brain to mitigate the seizures—and her miraculous recovery. But what deserves more recognition are her feats of athleticism and the unique mindset that has made her long and successful running career since then possible.

Her list of ultra-distance accolades is staggering, facilitated by a prestigious sponsorship with The North Face, which allows her to travel the globe running. She was the first woman to finish the Yukon Arctic Ultra 430-mile (692-km) race after winning the 300-mile (483-km) version outright the year before, towing a 45-pound supply sled across the ice-covered tundra in -50-degree (-45°C) conditions. She's finished in the top five at events like the 78-mile

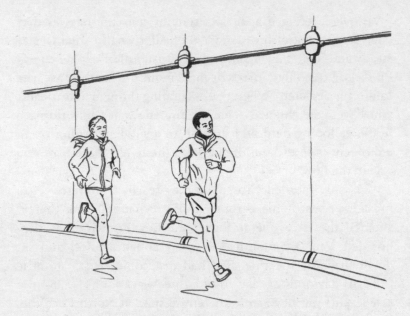

Having a sense of purpose in your running life brings greater meaning to everyday runs.

(125-km) Canadian Death Race in Edmonton, the Dances with Dirt 50 Mile (80 km) in Hell, Michigan, and the Hardrock 100 Mile (160 km) Endurance Run in Silverton, Colorado. She has traversed the treacherous Italian Dolomites, climbed South America's highest peak, trod through the jungle of the Philippines, run up the steps of the Great Wall of China, and negotiated the mountainous terrain of the Alps through France, Italy, and Switzerland.

On her Mountains-to-Sea Trail adventure, she ran and hiked as far as 62 miles (100 km) each day through all manner of weather, over the mud-soaked trails of the Blue Ridge Mountains and the treacherous, rocky overlooks of the Pisgah National Forest. She forded as many as 15 waist-deep streams in a single day before running toward the rolling Piedmont foothills. In just the first week, she trashed six pairs of running shoes.

On the morning of June 1, 2012, Van Deren climbed the last sand dune on the Outer Banks to Jockey's Ridge State Park, marking the end of her 1,175-mile (1,891-km) adventure, setting a new speed record of 22 days, 5 hours, and 3 minutes. When she reflects on that journey, she notes the various ways that the perfect running state materialized. There was the laser-focused, immersive awareness she experienced on that strip of Highway 12, but also a more serene attention on less harrowing days. She told me:

> *"On the harder stretches, I tried to let go of trying to control everything and allow myself to be in flow. I just welcomed what came my way and didn't fight against anything. And on easier terrain, I could just look ahead and go and I'd find a sense of flow and run in that state for miles. No matter the conditions, when I'm in flow, I'm totally focused on my footwork and using all my senses. I get into a rhythm as I'm listening to my feet and breathing. I'm not thinking about anything in particular, just hearing and feeling."*

To be sure, over the miles she's developed a unique proclivity for finding that special headspace. She said: "How do I find flow? First you have to train right, there's no shortcut. Second, you can't think about the outcome and must always stay in the moment. Third, you have to run with a sense of purpose and connection."

While you don't need to scale mountains or run for weeks on end to find it, Van Deren's story offers a revelatory example of how purpose can drive an intrinsic love for running, which thereby leads to a sense of running perfection. In this chapter we'll examine the ways purpose and identity in running can feed intrinsic motivation, which is inextricably linked to optimal experiences.

***

The Connection Between Intrinsic Motivation and Perfect Running

As was discussed in Chapter 3, when a person engages in an activity for intrinsic reasons—simply for the love of the activity itself—they are more likely to find that perfect running state. Similar to Csikszentmihalyi, Abraham Maslow identified intrinsic motivation as key to these transcendent experiences, finding that the people he studied all shared a love for a challenge. University of Quebec psychology professor Robert J. Vallerand refers to a concept that he calls "harmonious passion." He characterizes this as the motivation to engage in the work an activity like running requires simply because you take joy in the process itself.

This is antithetical to extrinsic motivation—the drive to do something out of a want for external rewards or accolades. While many runners may initially start running for extrinsic reasons as a means to an end—losing weight, finishing a marathon, scoring swag at a race—it won't sustain training over time. The day-to-day intentional practice of engaging in an activity that you truly enjoy is what cultivates continuity in happiness and motivation. "To get into the flow, I have to enjoy what I'm doing," Van Deren told me.

Interestingly, not only can intrinsic motivation help set the scene for the perfect running experience, perfect runs also have the potential to boost your enjoyment of running and enhance your motivation to train, thereby improving performance. It's what psychologists call a "virtuous cycle"—once you experience a perfect run, you desire more perfect runs, which drives you to continue training and seeking out bigger challenges. The by-product of that process is improved running prowess, optimal performance, and greater enjoyment.

Research out of the University of Zurich backs this up, showing that when first-time marathoners entered the flow state during their debut race, they experienced a heightened motivation to train, which translated into better subsequent performances. Even in the short term, studies have found that flow encourages runners to keep pushing when they experience setbacks. Entering that perfect headspace—or even having the knowledge that it exists—can be enough to carry you through a lackluster mile or low moment in the heat of competition. That persistence is key to good running.

Through their research, well-known psychologists Edward Deci and Richard Ryan found that three needs must be satisfied for intrinsic motivation to arise, something they dubbed the Self-Determination Theory. Other subsequent research has revealed that meeting these needs facilitates the flow experience:

1. Competency: You feel that you have the necessary wherewithal, skills, and control over influencing growth and success as a runner. Basically, you believe that if you put in effort, you'll see progress in your running.
2. Autonomy: You run because you have chosen to do so, not as a result of outside forces or obligation. It is important to feel that you have independent control over your participation in the sport.
3. Relatedness: You must feel a sense of connectedness and belonging within the sport. This can spring from relationships formed with running buddies or even the feeling of connection that is garnered participating in races and other running events.

Once these basic needs are met, you may be wondering what drives intrinsic motivation to endure over time. Studies suggest that interest plays a major role. Famed American philosopher and psychologist John Dewey long ago argued that when you're truly interested in an activity, some of the mental effort to complete the task falls away. In the case of running, a true love of the sport can feed this unforced sense of engagement, which is a major tenet of the perfect running experience.

Research backs up the fact that when a person experiences feelings of absorption, enjoyment, and enthusiasm when engaging in a specific task, as well as a sense of identity in relation to an activity, intrinsic motivation increases, thereby facilitating optimal experiences. Put simply, when you feel an emotional and personal connection to running, it reduces the cognitive load, allowing you to sustain engagement. These qualities not only help you persist through the tougher moments of a run, they are also important precursors to perfect running experiences. Van Deren's story aptly illustrates this. She told me this:

"I've always said that the recognition and attention that comes along with winning races and setting course records or doing something no one has ever done before only offers short-term satisfaction. To me, it has to have more purpose and meaning behind it, whether that means raising money for charity, helping to motivate someone, or give them hope. Course records and winning doesn't fulfill me. What fulfills me is helping others through my running. When you run with a sense of purpose, it's what is going to sustain you through the ups and downs of training. I love to run and be outside, but having purpose and connection beyond that is important."

Next, we will look at how finding purpose in your running and defining your identity as a runner can help build that sense of interest.

Discovering Purpose

As Van Deren alludes, if you hope to build intrinsic motivation and set the stage for more perfect running experiences, you must be able to identify a greater sense of purpose behind your training. When you step back and look at your running career thus far, ask yourself, is it the crossing of a race finish line and the cache of medals hanging on your wall that gives you a sense of meaning as a runner? Or is it the day-in and day-out training that contributes to that? While it can be easy to get preoccupied with distant objectives and accolades, researchers have discovered that happiness isn't a result of achieving big goals, but instead it comes from the ways we experience and interpret the chapters of our lives.

Indeed, this is evidenced by a long-term study out of Harvard University. The team of researchers interviewed men and women in diverse fields who exemplify a fulfilling life, discovering that the belief that success leads to fulfillment might be a backward assumption. Instead, their research reveals that pursuing fulfillment actually leads to success. When you feel an authentic affinity for running and approach it with intention, things like happiness, commitment, and achievement follow. Similarly, perfect running experiences can imbue your training with greater meaning, but the calculation goes both ways. By identifying a greater reason to run, you also set the stage for more perfect runs.

This should come as good news: In many cases you have the agency to cultivate and nurture happiness and the very quality of your life by gaining greater control of the inner workings of your mind. It doesn't mean that you don't pursue the big dreams, but it calls you to take the blinders off and pay attention to each passing mile on the road to getting there. In my first book, I introduce the concept of "True North Goals," which are the intentions you set for your running practice that have meaning beyond mileage, pounds, or pace. These objectives light the way toward self-improvement and greater contentment by emphasizing process over results.

Intentions are wholly separate from goals. Consider this example: If you decide to scale a mountain trail, your goal may be to run all the way to the summit. This is a useful objective because it provides inspiration to push through those lung-busting, quad-burning miles as you ascend to the top. Alternatively, an intention assists you in actually taking the necessary steps to reach your goal—it gives you a "why" for continuing to push to the top. While I will discuss the role of more traditional goal-setting methods in Chapter 5, consider some of the differences between goals and intentions:

- Goals are future-focused.
- Intentions are concerned with the present.
- Goals are aimed at a specific achievement or end game.
- Intentions are aimed at your lived experience in the moment.
- Goals are external accomplishments.
- Intentions are tied to your inner life and the way you interact with the world.

Exercise 4.1: What Drives You?

As you pinpoint your intentions, reflect on some of the reasons you run, as well as the benefits you gain from regular running. Here are some common intentions runners identify as important reasons to run:

- Greater mental and emotional balance
- More physical energy
- The chance to get out in nature
- The opportunity to reflect
- Modeling healthy behavior for family and children
- Exploring limits

Intentions guide you to live out your values through your running by putting an emphasis on the journey of training. Recent research reveals that taking time not only to reflect on and explore your personal values, but also to determine how they connect to your goals, has the power to improve performance beyond traditional goal-setting strategies. They remind you of the purpose behind your running practice and offer inspiration and motivation for daily training. To begin setting intentions or True North Goals, ask yourself the following questions:

- What matters to me most in life?
- What makes me happiest?
- What would I most like to let go of?
- How would I describe my best self?
- What do I feel grateful for?

Crafting a personal running mission statement is a great way to succinctly capture your True North Goals. This statement is centered on your running practice and can help keep you focused, inspired, and energized by giving you a clear sense of purpose behind your training.

Ask yourself:

- What is it about running that I'm drawn to?
- What do I hope to gain from running?
- What are my strengths as a runner?
- How does my running contribute to the greater good of my life, family, and/or the world around me?

Here's mine:

"To run for greater mental and physical balance in life. To carry forth the joy I gain from running into my other roles as a mother, wife, daughter, sister, friend, and writer. To create meaningful connections through running and share the love of movement with others."

Exercise 4.2: Using GPS to Craft Your Personal Running Mission Statement

Your running mission statement can assist you in prioritizing running when distractions in life interfere and threaten to pull you off the course of training. Remember to be flexible in crafting this statement and be open to making adjustments. Your sense of purpose when it comes to running may change depending on the stage of life you're in. Once you've reflected on what drives you to run, try writing your running mission statement. Some mission statements will be a single sentence, while others may be as long as a paragraph. Begin by listing the reasons you run before distilling them down into a statement. I suggest using this simple acronym to guide you: GPS.

G: Generate intentions—Wholly separate from goals, intentions are process-oriented and concerned with the greater purpose behind your running.

P: Prioritize passions—What is it that you truly love about running? Maybe it's the chance to get out in nature, be with your running comrades, spend time alone, or model healthy behavior for those around you. Try to identify things you love about running beyond the six-pack abs or the medal you get at the end of a race.

S: Synthesize intrinsic motivators—Distill your purpose and passions down to a single statement that paints a picture of your "why" when it comes to running.

Discovering Identity

One of my earliest memories is witnessing American Joan Benoit Samuelson win the first women's Olympic marathon in 1984 on the streets of Los Angeles. I watched the inaugural event on a black-and-white television in the living room of our home in Minneapolis with my dad, a marathoner and running fan. At just 1¼ miles (2 km) into the race, the pack of 50 or so runners had already exceeded any distance ever run by women on the Olympic stage. Although I was too young to understand the significance at the time, this was a momentous race that was part of a wave of new opportunities for women and girls in sports from which I would reap the benefits.

From the early miles of the race, Joan went out hard, running far ahead of the pack. The commentators chalked it up to inexperience, surmising that New York City Marathon legend Grete Waitz of Norway would handily reel her in. The rest of the pack stuck with Waitz, but Joan pushed by herself up front the entire way. When she appeared on the other side of the dark tunnel leading into the L.A. Coliseum—the first to enter the stadium—she had one full lap around the track to go. Urged on by a roaring crowd, she waved her white painter's cap and appeared to glide effortlessly over the final meters of the race, throwing up her arms as she crossed the finish line. Back in Minneapolis, my dad and I jumped around the living room hollering "Joanie! Joanie!"

Although I was very young, that race made a real impression on me. That day I saw Joan Benoit Samuelson set the pace and write her own narrative without uttering a word. In interviews since, she has talked about how you can live out your values and goals and tell your story through your running – that a true passion for running breaks down barriers in your mind and allows you to forge your own authentic path. This is important because research demonstrates that people who pursue an activity for the sheer love of the task itself, without concern for what others think, are more prone to encounter optimal experiences. Examining your running narrative—or cultivating one if it doesn't already exist—can help facilitate personal interest in and a greater connection to the sport, paving the way for perfect running.

To do this, you must reflect on whether your stated intentions for training match up with your day-to-day running. The ways in which you arrange the plot points of your running life into a narrative play a major role in shaping who you are as a runner. Your narrative arc—the stories you tell yourself about how and why you became a runner, how and why you continue to run, the ways in which you see yourself as a runner, and where you see yourself going as a runner—all shape current reality.

Exercise 4.3: Visualizing the Runner You Want to Be

Identifying a reason behind your running is all about seeing yourself as the runner you want to be. A great way to solidify this image is through the use of imagery. In fact, experts suggest that for athletes, imagery exercises can play an important role in prompting the positive psychological states that set the stage for flow. Studies even demonstrate that visualization can impact performance in dynamic ways by amplifying the flow experience.

So how do you employ visualization to form a solid image of the runner you want to be? Start with this simple exercise:

- Sit in a quiet, comfortable place and close your eyes.
- Take five deep breaths and allow your body a few moments to relax.
- Try to create a detailed image in your mind of an upcoming performance scenario, like the start line of a race or warming up for a workout.
- Take in the sights, sounds, feelings, and smells around you. Work on employing your senses to establish a picture of the scene. What's the weather like? Who else is there? How do your legs feel? What are you wearing?
- Imagine the gun firing at the beginning of a race or clicking your watch at the start of a workout. Take a few minutes to watch the scene unfold. Again, continue to take note of the sights, sounds, smells, and physical sensations you might experience.
- If you get distracted and find your mind wandering at any point in this exercise, simply take note and redirect to where you left off.

- Work on maintaining positive images throughout, seeing yourself running tall and strong. You can even reflect on the positive self-talk you might use along the way.
- As the run comes to an end, see yourself finishing with strength and confidence. Imagine how that would feel in real time. What do your legs and lungs feel like? How are your energy levels? What about your mood?
- Take five more slow, deep breaths as you focus on that image of yourself. Repeat this exercise in the coming days to further solidify this picture in your mind.

In narrative psychology, a person's story doesn't just consist of the details and events of their life, but the ways that person takes those details and events and integrates them to make sense and meaning. This is how we form our identities as runners—we choose which things to include and emphasize in our narrative, as well as the ways we want to frame them. The story of you as a runner can take widely diverging paths depending on how you frame the episodes of your running career. Interestingly, the lens through which you see yourself may have developed as early as adolescence, making it quite rigid. If you dubbed yourself a poor athlete back in high school P.E. class, it can be a real challenge to shake that sense of yourself. On the other hand, if your entire identity is wrapped up in being a runner, that narrowness can cause issues too.

The problem with these lenses is that they often shade out your ability to see yourself in a new light—to grow, change, and develop. In mindfulness circles, the idea of the "beginner's mind" is all about viewing yourself and the world around you with fresh eyes in order to be open to novel discoveries. Indeed, there is evidence to suggest that being open to fresh ideas and characterizations can be a boon to health and well-being and as was discussed in Chapter 3, this openness can also expedite perfect running experiences.

Exercise 4.4: Story Editing

In the same way a writer might edit an essay, so too can a runner revise his or her own personal story by interpreting experiences in new ways. In the case of a negative or unproductive inner narrative, one way to do this editing is through what is called cognitive restructuring. This is a method by which you leverage facts against irrational worries and beliefs. Try the following:

Take note of your cognitive distortions. For instance, if you notice you tend to make negative predictions leading up to races or big workouts, work on simply noticing when your mind forms those thoughts. Maybe prior to a race, you catch yourself thinking: "I know I can't handle the hot weather today and I'm totally going to crash and burn." Then ask yourself a series of questions to confront that distorted belief:

• How else might I think about this and reframe this situation leading up to the race?
• What's the worst that could happen in this race?
• What's the best that could happen in this race?
• What's the most likely thing to happen?

Recent research also reveals that your inner narrative and beliefs have a tangible effect on potential and performance. One study out of Stanford University conducted genetic testing on participants to identify gene variants that influence a person's capacity for exercise. They also had each do a running time trial on a treadmill to measure endurance. Then they randomly split the group into two, telling one group that they had the variant of a gene that makes a person fatigue more easily. The other was told they had the gene variant that was linked to higher endurance. Since they were randomly divided, some of the participants received accurate results and others didn't.

After the revelation of their supposed genetic results, they had the participants hop on the treadmill for another time trial. Interestingly, participants who thought they had poor endurance genes didn't run as far or as long. They had reduced lung capacity and their bodies didn't process carbon dioxide as efficiently—all as a result of believing they weren't genetically endowed with natural endurance prowess. Those who were told they had the endurance genes ran longer, regardless of whether they actually had those genes or not. Put simply, the information supposedly gathered from the genetic testing significantly affected these runners' inner narratives, which actually altered their physiology.

A running narrative doesn't just cover the main events of your running existence—workouts you've logged, the times you've run, and the races you've finished. It communicates over the course of training what was important and why. The arc of a runner's story offers both continuity and identity. A positive-leaning narrative with a strong protagonist has a way of creating meaning and coherence out of the episodes of your running life. When your inner narrative involves a clear story regarding who you are as a runner, integrating ideas about where you've been and where you hope to go, the potential exists to find greater purpose.

What runners say

Of the runners I surveyed, many pointed to factors related to their personal running narrative and the ways they related to inner and outer expectations that helped them get into that perfect running headspace or, conversely, detracted from it. Here's what some said:

"The biggest flow trigger for me is when I am excited for my workout and feel mentally good about life."
Michael G., 38, North Bend, OR

"I keep things simple. I have become rather minimalist with regards to my kit. I used to follow standard advice carrying backpacks, drinks, and food, but it dawned on me that no matter which direction I run from my house, even through the wild countryside, I am never more than 5 miles from a shop, garage, or pub. So I tend to just go out in the bare essentials to stay safe and that makes me feel really good, which I believe helps me reach flow. I also don't pay attention to the weather, I used to fuss about what to wear if it's raining/cold/foggy/sunny. Now I just use common sense."

Phil B., 55, Basingstoke, Hampshire, UK

"Thinking and reflecting on positive thoughts is important, especially an upcoming race you feel good about or a good race that you just ran."

Michael P., 42, California, PA

"For sure, the 'thinky brain' can be a real limiter to finding the flow state. When your brain says things like, 'you should be running faster,' 'you're getting passed by a nine-year-old,' 'you look fat in these running shorts,' or 'you have awkward running form,' it blocks you from just running. Taking the ego out of running is huge when it comes to finding flow. Taking away 'should be' is important: I should be running x:xx/mile or I'm not a good runner. I should be running x:xx/mile or I'm not doing the workout correctly. I should be passing that guy/lady/kid. Just start out easy and let the run come to you."

John G., 40, Philadelphia, PA

"Feeling tired mentally and/or physically definitely keeps me from getting in the zone. If you have loads of time pressures when going for a run, that doesn't help at all either."

Sarah E., 49, Hereford, UK

"Getting caught up in the highs and lows of running distracts from getting in the zone. When I let my highs get too high and lows get too low, I start to lose focus."

Randi B., 35, Dallas, TX

"I find that simply being fit and rested leads to this feeling. And, in turn, one's mental state continues to improve when you're running in the zone."

Tom D., 58, Sydney, Australia

"Pressure, unreasonable expectations, and a busy mind that doesn't let you focus and relax all interrupt flow."

Jason F., 35, Denver, CO

If you hope to cultivate more perfect running experiences, you want intentions and narrative to align. Keep in mind that while a positive running narrative helps set the stage for the perfect running experience, when you are actually in that headspace, that inner monologue deactivates. While many things can influence your running narrative, there are four main psychological constructs that affect it in important ways: Self-awareness, self-belief, self-talk, and self-compassion.

1. Self-Awareness: The ways you monitor and interpret yourself and your inner world

Self-awareness helps you recognize the things you tell yourself about yourself. This is key to determining whether there is coherence between the runner you are and the runner you want to be. A keen awareness of your consciousness can enable you to function with greater authenticity, as well as assist you in gaining a better understanding of your "true self" as a runner. Mindfulness is inextricably linked to self-awareness because it encourages attention to be paid to the emotions, attitudes, and thoughts that influence your inner world, as well as the way you interact with the outer world. Honing a strong sense of self-awareness is essential to creating continuity in your narrative.

Exercise 4.5: Practicing Body Awareness

Just as we have long known that our mental weather can affect the way we feel physically, the science of embodied cognition also suggests that our bodies can influence cognition. For example, slouching can decrease a person's sense of self-esteem, while standing in an expansive and confident pose can make a person feel more powerful. This underscores the inextricable relationship between body and mind and the ways that greater awareness of both can influence one another. As you begin to pay more attention to your thoughts and emotions, also work to identify the accompanying physical response. Anxiety at the start line of a race may lead to tight shoulders or vice versa. An open and present-focused mind may make you feel more relaxed physically or vice versa. As you begin to pair thoughts and emotions with physical responses, you'll gain a greater sense of awareness in the moment, which can assist in strengthening a more productive running narrative.

---

2. Self-belief: The things you believe about yourself

In the 1970s, Stanford psychologist Albert Bandura showed that when a person believed they were equipped with the necessary skills to meet a challenge and succeed—what he called self-efficacy—their motivation to do so, in turn, increased. Self-belief is concerned with how you perceive your potential as a runner—the core feelings and ideas you harbor about yourself. These feelings and beliefs are ultimately constructed or eroded through your experiences as a runner and the ways you interpret those experiences. A healthy sense of self-belief signals a growth mindset—you have confidence in your potential to develop and progress. This assists a runner in setting realistic but increasingly challenging goals, which may then result in more perfect running experiences, something that will be discussed further in Chapter 5. Self-belief plays a major role in whether you see yourself as a strong protagonist in your running narrative.

Exercise 4.6: The Power of *Yet*

Self-belief is largely about interpretation. Do you interpret lackluster workouts and missed race goals as failures or stepping stones in your development as a runner? To flip the script on an inner voice that lacks self-belief, I like to employ the word "yet." Try adding "yet" to the following types of statement next time you catch yourself in a crisis of confidence.

- "I can't do this ... yet"
- "I'm not fit enough ... yet"
- "I'm not capable of that ... yet"

---

3. Self-talk: The way you communicate with yourself

When you are out running, is your inner script positive or negative? Many runners tend to be hard on themselves, harboring a merciless inner critic. Unfortunately, that negative narrator signals a skewed interpretation of self and has a way of warping and flattening the main character in your running narrative. Not only do we know that positive self-talk is essential to constructing an authentic and motivational inner narrative, it can also help boost performance.

Exercise 4.7: Tuning in to Your Inner Voice

Learning to identify the nature of your self-talk is the first step in determining whether your inner voice is contributing to a satisfying running career or eroding it. Devote your next easy run to getting a handle on the tenor of that narrator. As you begin to run, take note of the thoughts that pop into your head. How are you talking to yourself? Some of the thoughts may be neutral or totally unrelated to running, so pay special attention to those that are about running itself.

As these thoughts come into your mind, attach a mental label to them. For instance, if you're running up a hill, you may think: "Wow, that strength training I've been doing is really paying off, I feel great!" The label you could attach: Encouragement. On the flip side, as you round out the final miles of your workout, you think: "I was way slower today than I should have been." The label you could attach: Criticism. Over the course of a single or several runs, you'll begin to get a read on whether your inner voice trends positive or negative. While no runner will be 100 percent positive all the time, simply understanding your thought patterns and what is productive and what isn't can help guide you in welcoming or working to steer away from certain types of thinking.

---

4. Self-compassion: The ways you judge yourself

Nonjudgmental awareness is a key tenet of mindfulness and perfect running. A big part of this is the way you judge yourself and whether you observe yourself, your thoughts, and your actions with kindness and curiosity or harsh criticism. A judgmental inner commentary not only signals a disconnect with your running mission statement, it will also serve as an unproductive distraction during workouts and races. While we all fall short of our ambitions sometimes, research demonstrates that being able to forgive yourself with a sense of kindness allows you to more quickly return to the task at hand. Indeed, self-compassion has been shown to increase perseverance among athletes. Similarly, other studies suggest that self-compassion and exercise motivation are linked by helping you get over failures and disappointments with greater expedience, thereby allowing you to redouble your efforts and get back to training. Look for more on self-compassion in Chapter 9.

Exercise 4.8: Socratic Questioning

From an early age, we are taught The Golden Rule: To treat others the way you want to be treated. Somewhere along the line, though, many of us stop treating ourselves with kindness and forgiveness. Instead of considering a workout or race that didn't turn out the way we hoped as a learning experience, we ruthlessly chastise ourselves. While disappointment is healthy and normal, getting down on yourself for days and weeks isn't productive. This is where "Socratic questioning" comes in. This exercise simply calls you to ask yourself, "Would I talk to a running partner or friend this way?" If not, you might consider showing yourself more compassion. This approach has been shown to reduce depressive thinking because it guides you to consider the validity of negative thinking and expand your view to a broader perspective.

Now that we've covered the foundational step of building an authentic sense of purpose into your running practice, Chapter 5

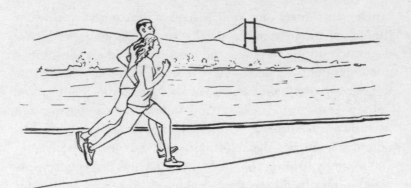

Establishing a positive narrative is essential to perfect running.

will cover the importance of planning. From establishing a running routine, to setting goals, to choosing a training plan, all of these steps are important on the road to discovering more perfect running experiences.

Practices in Perfection

- When a runner is intrinsically motivated, they run out of a pure love for the sport. This must be present for the perfect running state to arise.
- Identifying purpose and setting intentions can help build genuine interest in running. Crafting a personal running mission statement is a good way to succinctly capture those intentions.
- Defining your identity as a runner through narrative storytelling can also boost interest. The four psychological constructs that can most significantly influence that narrative are self-awareness, self-belief, self-talk, and self-compassion.

CHAPTER 5

PLANNING

*"The flow state is an elevated level of awareness. My
mind is totally engaged and everything besides the task
at hand is a blur."*

THE ATMOSPHERE BUZZED with electricity at the start of the
2014 Boston Marathon. As nearly 36,000 nervous runners huddled
in nearby tents and jumped up and down trying to stay warm and
relaxed, the announcer urged them to "Take back that finish line!"
Simultaneously, over a million fans—nearly twice the number
that usually come out to watch the race on Patriot's Day—flooded
the streets of Beantown to support the athletes. With everyone in
a heightened state of awareness beyond the normal race reverie,
more than 3,500 police officers patrolled the city, Blackhawk
helicopters flew overhead, the national guard was on alert, and
hundreds of security cameras recorded along the course.

This marked the first anniversary of the Boston Marathon
bombing that killed four people and injured more than 260
others. The morning was marked by an air of solemnity, but also
resilience. The mantra "Boston Strong" was everywhere. Runners,
race officials, fans, and locals alike came together to show that the
determination and sense of community that characterized this
century-old event was stronger than the terror inflicted upon the
city the year prior.

The 2009 winner of the New York City Marathon and silver medalist at the Athens Olympics, Meb Keflezighi, stood among the other elite runners at the start line. Reporters, however, were largely focused on American Ryan Hall, the only runner to have run a sub-2:05 marathon (2:04.58 at the 2011 Boston Marathon) and the likely Kenyan or Ethiopian winners. The event was traditionally dominated by runners who hailed from those countries—they'd captured 24 out of the past 30 Boston Marathon titles.

Meb held the 15th fastest personal best among the elite field that day, 2:09:08 run at the 2012 London Olympics. He was older than most of the other elite competitors, just two weeks shy of his 39th birthday, and had recently lost a prestigious sponsorship. Most assumed that his best running days were behind him. None of this concerned him, though. He'd been visualizing this race for an entire year. At the 2013 event, Meb sat in the grandstands at the finish line in a state of awe and inspiration. Just moments before a bomb blasted that very area, he'd left for the press room. It was that tragic event that led him to set a goal to return in pursuit of the title.

A few days prior, I'd flown into Boston with my husband for the race. He qualified to run but, hampered by an injury, decided to spectate. I'd run the race before and had also sat in the press room alternating between watching it on the big screen and standing at the finish line. I decided that I wanted to experience race day from a fan's perspective that year—to see what "Boston Strong" was all about. I joined my husband and some friends who lived in the city and we hustled around by train to various points along the course.

It was at mile 8 (13 km) that Meb and fellow American Josphat Boit gapped the rest of the elite field. By the halfway point, they'd built up a 30-second lead. In post-race interviews, the other top runners would report feeling unthreatened by Meb's move at the time. Most were focused on defending champion Lelisa Desisa, waiting to see what he would do. After all, the second half of

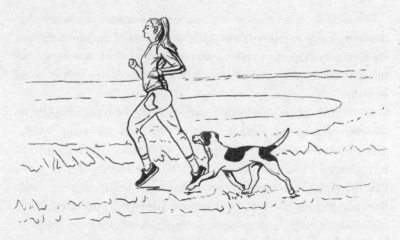

Being intentional about your running can contribute to more satisfying runs.

Boston is notoriously more challenging than the first, so they all figured they'd eventually reel him back in. Meanwhile, at 15.5 miles (25 km), Meb found himself all alone up front. Later he would tell me, "I can't even recall crossing the halfway marker. I was in a state of absolute focus. It's a beautiful thing."

By the time Meb reached the infamous Heartbreak Hill, about 22 miles (35 km) into the race, many still discounted the possibility of an American win. In transit to the finish, I checked my phone. On social media there were reports that Meb's lead had shrunk to just eight seconds with Wilson Chebet of Kenya in hot pursuit. Meb ran 5:00 minutes flat for the 25th mile, looking over his shoulder several times to judge how much of a lead he held. While his pace hadn't slowed, Chebet's quickened.

Pushing past crowds and security barriers, we arrived just in time to see Meb turn left on Boylston Street, legging it down the final .35-mile (.56-km) stretch of the race. He'd maintained and widened his lead over Chebet. The crowd was deafening. American flags waved and tears were shed. Improbably, Meb became the first American man to win Boston in more than three decades.

In his book *26 Marathons*, he wrote that something clicked that day to produce a sense of flow amid moments of intense suffering. He told me: "The flow state is an elevated level of awareness. My mind is totally engaged and everything besides the task at hand is a blur."

At the finish line, Meb was crowned with the traditional laurel wreath reserved for winners of the race. His bib read "MEB," along with the names of the people who were killed during the bombings the year prior. It was those people and the 2013 tragedy that drove Meb to originally set a goal to win that day. Even with the tremendous pressure he'd put on himself, coupled with the dismissal of his prospects, he was calm and relaxed from the start, reminding himself to work on controlling only what was in his purview and to let go of the rest.

In his training, he committed to a big goal, but then set it aside and focused on the daily work that was required to get there. This process-focused mindset is what paved the path toward his perfect run that day. Whether you're gunning for a win at one of the most prestigious races in the world or a personal best in your local 5K, this experience is within reach for every runner. This chapter is all about how to set smart goals and put your training on a path toward perfection.

***

Determining Goals

When it comes to maintaining the motivation to engage in training and practice, goals provide a blueprint for where you want to go and help to direct your psychic energy and attention in purposeful and specific ways, which also fuels commitment to training. As we've learned from foundational flow research, a balance between your fitness and skill level and the challenge you hope to pursue must be struck if you hope to create the right conditions for more perfect running experiences.

Research backs this up: A report published by Harvard Business School suggests that when goals are too ambitious, they can be self-defeating and only serve to reduce motivation. At the same time, trivial goals just signal that you don't trust your own potential. Underselling yourself leads to apathy and stagnation in training. Indeed, a willingness to set high goals and take calculated risks, particularly risking failure, can set you up to experience more perfect runs. Think about it: If you assume you will be able to run a 5K in under 30 minutes and then you go out and do that, you risk very little. You've created no room to stretch your potential. When failure is a possibility, there's a certain thrill that comes from achieving that goal.

Exercise 5.1: Goal Setting Reflection

Before setting and pursuing a goal, it's worth taking a little time to ask yourself a few questions to make sure it serves the purpose you want it to serve. Here are some examples:

- Is this something I'll enjoy doing?
- What will I need to sacrifice to achieve this goal?
- How will I feel when I accomplish it?
- Are there other goals that are more important to me?

People report being happiest when they are in pursuit of something that challenges them, but is still within reach. That's where the perfect running channel exists. The struggle to pursue lofty goals and overcome the barriers to them sows the seeds for perfect running experiences. No matter what you're training for, a runner's journey is more marathon than sprint. Different types of goals serve as signposts that lead you in a desired direction toward a specific endgame. As such, I like to split goals into three separate categories: Long-term goals, short-term goals, and micro goals.

Long-term goals

According to some experts, we have evolved to go after long-term goals because our hunter-gatherer forebears had to pursue prey even when the odds weren't in their favor. Long-term goals often involve a major race some months down the line. Whether it's a 5K or a marathon, having a race on the calendar helps guide training and provide structure. Another common long-term goal is weight loss. While pounds will be shed over the course of training, that end goal on the scale can serve to drive you for many months.

Short-term goals

Short-term goals usually have to do with a specific workout or training goal. This could be as simple as challenging yourself to run a new route or distance at a certain pace. Or it could be to add an extra interval on to your speed workout. Maybe it just means not walking on a run. Research shows that when mice adeptly navigate a maze, achieving smaller objectives on the way to an ultimate goal (finishing the maze), their bodies release dopamine, which is associated with motivation. Experts posit that it works the same way with humans. By setting short-term goals, you encourage a state of continuous development.

Micro goals

I like to call the goals that come up mid-run, on-the-fly, "micro goals." This could be something as simple as challenging yourself to hold a specific pace for another mile or continue to run to the next stop light. In the habit literature, these are called "small wins." They are small accomplishments along the way that aid motivation and belief in the possibility of larger "wins." B.J. Fogg, a researcher of human behavior at Stanford University, constructed a behavioral model that suggests that a person's move to action is dependent on both motivation and skill to execute a given task. If you overestimate your abilities, you're likely to burn out, but if you increase the challenge little by little, small wins add up to lasting and significant progress and consistency. The takeaway for runners is that there are no shortcuts. Choosing to go after even the smallest micro goals can elicit real and discernable progress.

As they begin to conceive these different "sized" goals, I direct athletes I coach to reflect on a goal-setting approach borrowed from the business world. This is known as S.M.A.R.T. goals, which stands for Specific, Measurable, Achievable, Relevant, and Time-bound. Each of your goals, whether they be short, long, or micro, should fit into this framework. And remember to jot them down as you go through this process—research shows that you're more likely to stay committed when you've put them in writing:

- **Specific** Set up a time and a place for your goals to be achieved. Signing up for a race or identifying an event for which you want to lose weight are good examples.
- **Measurable** Instead of setting a nebulous goal, like "I want to be a faster runner," go into a bit more detail. It could be, "I want to run a two-hour personal best in the half marathon" or "I want to finish my first 5K."
- **Achievable** Choose a goal that pushes you, but isn't totally out of your reach.
- **Relevant** Your goals should sprout from your own personal ambitions, not something your running buddy wants to do.
- **Time-bound** Keep your training on a time table. Signing up for a race is a great way to accomplish this.

A Reminder About Enjoying the Journey: Skill development and mounting fitness often necessitate adjustment of goals. While a 4:30-hour marathon might have once been your long-term goal, maybe now you're capable of a 4:15. Mindfully monitoring progress is vital to avoid missing out on reaching your true potential. At the same time, as we seek to achieve new and higher goals, mounting expectations can make running satisfaction feel unattainable. This is the danger of setting big goals—sometimes the pressure to achieve becomes more important than the journey of training.

When we can enjoy the present moment and whatever challenge is directly in front of us, we are more likely to find contentment in running. Goals are important—they serve as vital sources of motivation and direction—but it's not the only reason to run. Check your mindset every now and again to make sure you haven't put on the blinders in pursuit of your long-term goals.

* * *

Selecting a Training Plan

Most of us need some sort of training plan to stay on track and motivated toward our goals. While going into detail about training specifics is beyond the scope of this book, it's worth mentioning the basics. Those perfect runs only happen when you're implementing strategic training—the training that we've learned works thanks to our running forefathers and mothers—so taking time to decide your course of action is well worth the investment.

Smart training programs are important because they provide a framework within which a runner can test limits and stay on track toward a goal. Whether it's a 5k or a marathon and you're a newbie or a veteran, there's something for every runner. With that said, if you aren't training for a specific event, you may be looking for something a bit less regimented. That's okay too. You may still want a general training plan mapped out to help you get out the door each day, but one that allows for more flexibility.

Components of a Successful Training Program: While every training program is different, especially those that are tailored to the individual, there are several guiding principles that will underscore any smart training philosophy. Make sure your plan does the following:

- Addresses overall health and fitness
- Prevents overtraining and burnout
- Includes recovery days and easy runs
- Integrates a variety of training tactics

Remember that checking with your doctor is always advisable when starting a training plan, especially if you're a new runner. No matter your goals, intentions, and circumstances, taking a tailored approach is key. The right training plan can go a long way toward cultivating more perfect running experiences. Here are some of the key elements of any training plan to take note of before committing to a particular course of action.

- **Mileage**: If you haven't been running at all, be conservative in your initial buildup. With good reason, many beginner programs combine running and walking to help develop fitness before throwing you into full-time running. If you've been running already, most coaches suggest building about 10 percent per week. That means if you ran 20 miles (32 km) last week, this week you would run 22 miles (35 km) and so forth. No matter what your starting point, a gradual build in mileage and intensity is vital to avoiding injury.

- **Length of program**: The majority of running programs last somewhere between 12 and 30 weeks. If you're working toward a race, be sure that the program you choose gives you enough time to complete the entire training protocol.

- **Level of difficulty**: It can be hard to know how high to shoot when selecting a training program. Most online options offer some guidance, but it often also involves trial and error. Consider your current fitness and your goal race and pace when zeroing in on a plan and be open to adjusting when necessary. Remember, matching your skill and fitness level with training is essential to unlocking more of those perfect runs.

- **Weekly schedule**: Some training programs have runners exercising three days a week and others six. Consider the time commitment you'll be able to afford running when choosing a plan.

- **Variety**: We all love our routines, but good training plans will encourage you to vary things like terrain, pace, route, and setting. Workouts should involve the various energy systems in calculated ways as well. Some of the most common types of workouts to include are as follows: Intervals, tempo, long runs, easy runs, hills, cross-training, strength, and flexibility/mobility.

- **Rest and recovery**: Rest and recovery days are essential for allowing training adaptations to take hold. Even the pros report running upward of 80 percent of their miles at an easy or moderate pace. What's more, they are as committed to rest and recovery as they are to training itself.

Should You Hire a Coach?: Recruiting the help of a coach can take your running to the next level. There's no denying the benefits of the individualized attention, guidance, and knowledge that an expert can provide. When it comes to cost, there are a number of options, from online advice to in-person one-on-one attention. Start by scouring the internet and researching coaches in your area and consider scheduling an initial meeting to see if your agendas match up.

* * *

The Big Picture

Keep in mind that your physiology is affected by the neurobiological context of training. Put simply, training doesn't occur in a vacuum. Stress from other areas of life will affect how you feel on a run, as well as how your body adapts to training. On cellular and systemic levels, adaptation is influenced by stress in ways that are hard to predict.

Consider the example of load limits on the roof of a building. It all has to do with physics. The roof has to be able to support a temporary load of, say, a team of roofers or, where I live, several feet of snow. It also has to withstand "uplift load," which occurs when a gust of wind hits the exterior sides and disperses upward and downward energy. If you're building a house, it is important for the contractor to have knowledge of both physics and engineering and then consult a building code book to determine load limits depending on the span of the roof's rafters, lumber dimensions, and wood species. Being able to pinpoint just how much stress you can place on the roof becomes a simple equation. The roof's load or carrying capacity doesn't change based on the roof's mood or what it was doing earlier in the day. If it did, it would be nearly impossible to build a proper roof. A highly anxious roof might cave at the first sign of snow flurries, while a more confident roof may be able to withstand a wicked blizzard.

Runners, on the other hand, face this issue all the time. There are many variables in life that can increase stress—a tough boss, relationship problems, financial issues. Navigating them all effectively is a challenge and figuring out how to factor that stress into training can feel next to impossible. Since a building code book can't help you put together your training the same way it can help you construct a roof, learning to listen to your body within the larger context of your life becomes imperative.

What runners say

Many of the runners I spoke with about the perfect running experience said that stress outside of running was a sure way to eliminate their ability to reach that next-level headspace. Here's what some had to say:

"Outside stress can definitely interfere, but at times it's such a great stress reliever that even when things are tough in the real world, you can shut thoughts out and run amazingly. For the flow state runs you need to be 100 percent focused on running, not thinking about other things."

Sarah E., 49, Hereford, UK

"Dwelling on a bad day of training, a busy work schedule, or fretting about pain or soreness keeps me from finding flow."

Michael P., 42, California, TX

"Low stress outside of running and coming into workouts mentally fresh definitely helps me get to that place. Also, coming into workouts relatively rested, not low on sleep, sets you up to tap in to the zone more easily."

Lindsay L., 39, Harrisburg, PA

"Stress can definitely get in the way. We are all human and no matter how much we want to forget our issues, sometimes our brains won't let us. I do still firmly believe that running is the best natural antidepressant for me though."

Phil B., 55, Basingstoke, Hampshire, UK

"Having too many negative thoughts in my head gets in the way, whether it is stress related to the workout, life, or work."

Michael G., 38, North Bend, OR

"Outside life stress is probably the biggest limiter. It tends to keep my mind from staying focused and getting into the zone."

Carl L., 38, Atlanta, GA

"Stress at work can affect getting into a calm and relaxed state on a run. Although running often helps to dampen the stress, the run is not as fluid as when I'm less stressed and more relaxed. I think that the more thoughts that are going through your head, the less able you are to concentrate on tuning in to your breathing and stride, which I know for me is key to getting in the zone."

Amanda, H., 48, Droitwich, UK

Entire books have been written about the logistics involved in training. That's not this book. The focus here is on the psychological factors that are amenable to perfect running experiences. With that said, it's worth noting some of the logistical aspects of training that must be addressed if you hope to achieve more of those perfect runs. Keeping these things in

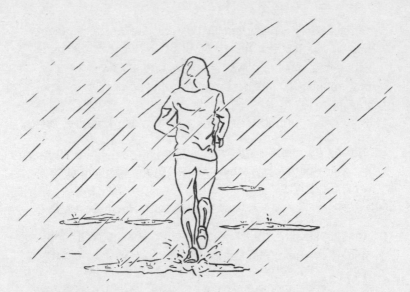

The quality of your runs is often influenced by other areas of life.

mind will help bolster performance as you progress through your training plan.

- **Hydration**: One study found that proper hydration could improve 10K times by an average of a whole minute, while others have demonstrated that even a small decrement in hydration status can decrease performance. To keep your hydration levels up, work to drink mostly water throughout the day, supplementing with some sports drinks, especially when it's hot. Check with a doctor or coach for specifics pertaining to your situation.

- **Nutrition**: Running nutrition involves eating enough calories, the right calories, and taking in calories at the right times. There are plenty of online calculators to help you figure out what and how much to consume, but keep in mind that as your mileage goes up, so will your caloric needs. Running on too little fuel is a recipe for lackluster training and racing. While every runner's dietary needs will differ, getting the right balance of carbohydrates, protein, and fats will aid performance and recovery.

- **Fueling**: If you are running over an hour, you'll need to form a strategy for fueling and hydration on the run. Your plan should be highly individualized—some runners can stomach just about anything, while others must be quite selective. The key here is to practice your nutritional strategy well ahead of any scheduled events, so you know what works.

- **Sleep**: Sleep is essential to good running for a number of reasons. First and foremost, high-volume protein synthesis occurs while you sleep, which leads to muscle repair following hard workouts. While a solid eight hours is generally recommended, researchers suggest that more— upward of ten hours—can improve athletic performance. While you might not have that kind of time to devote to getting shut-eye, you can still work to get adequate rest, especially during periods of intense training.

- **Environment**: Mixing up terrain and training environments can help keep you engaged in training. When choosing where to run, first consider safety. Avoiding highly secluded locations is often a good idea, but you also want to make sure you aren't constantly dodging traffic. In addition, work on identifying routes that you actually look forward to. Nice scenery and the company of other runners passing in a park can boost mood and performance on the run. If you tend to lose yourself in perfect runs, be mindful about maintaining some level of awareness of your surroundings.

- **Timing**: The time of day that you run will depend on when you have free time. If you have any flexibility, keep in mind daylight and weather. Running during daylight hours tends to be a safer option. What's more, extreme cold and heat might guide when is best to get in your run. If you stick to a regular schedule and run around the same time each day, it can make planning easier.

Our understanding of the physiological aspects of stress is being illuminated by new research, which points to the importance of looking at physiological, emotional, and environmental circumstances when charting training plans and predicting training responses. In short, there's no one-size-fits-all training plan and even when you do put together a tailored schedule, adjustments often need to be made in response to unforeseen stress in other areas of life. Even cutting-edge technological devices can't factor in life stress the way simple self-awareness can. This is why a purposeful, process-focused approach to training, which will be discussed further in the next chapter, is so vital.

Practices in Perfection

- When your fitness and skillset are well matched to the challenge of a workout or race, you're more likely to encounter the perfect running experience.
- Goals should push you to reach your full potential, but still need to be realistic.
- As you reflect on your running ambitions, work to set long-term, short-term, and micro goals.
- Your training plan should be tailored to your intentions, goals, fitness, and skillset.
- When it comes to smart training, the big picture is important to consider. Physiological, emotional, environmental, and circumstantial stress from other areas of life can affect training and necessitate adjustments.

CHAPTER 6
PROCESS

"It's so easy to get stuck in a rut; it's so hard to adventure out. But if you don't try different things, you don't learn much, and you have little chance to discover your own perfect-flow race."

ON APRIL 19, 1968, Amby Burfoot and Bill Clark ran stride for stride as they moved up, over, and down the grueling section of Newton hills along the Boston Marathon course. This punishing stretch culminates at Heartbreak Hill at mile 20 (32 km). This is where Burfoot, a 6-foot tall, 130-pound, 21-year-old college senior, decided to make his move. Clark, a former track star and Marine lieutenant, was known for his strong finishing speed and this, Burfoot decided, would be his chance to gain some distance on his challenger.

He unleashed a burst of speed and strength as he began his ascent up Heartbreak Hill, driving hard with heavy arms and legs. The 70-degree (21°C) midday sun beat down and sweat poured off his face and stung his eyes. With no water stops along the course, his mouth was parched and his throat burned. As he crested the hill, his vision narrowed. He looked down at the asphalt in front of him to see not one, but two shadows moving in tandem. Despite his best efforts, he couldn't seem to shake Clark.

Burfoot set a goal of winning the Boston Marathon years earlier. He started running as a junior in high school in Groton, Connecticut, in the early 1960s. He immediately took to the sport. In a 2004 *Runner's World* article, he wrote about his first encounter with the runner's high as a youngster. Training near his childhood home one "perfect" October day, he recalled the smells from the nearby cider mill hanging in the air. Twigs and leaves crunched underfoot as he slipped into a "timeless" state, feeling almost as if he were floating.

During his early years in the sport, Burfoot's head was filled with tales of legendary Boston Marathon history by his high school coach and two-time Olympian, John J. Kelley, who'd won the race in 1957. Burfoot himself first toed the line in Hopkinton in 1965, joining 358 other runners. He ended up finishing 25th and in 1967 returned to finish 17th. After that, he redoubled his efforts in training, running upward of 175 miles (280 km) some weeks in preparation for the 1968 event.

Things began to click in a unique way and he felt fresher, faster, and stronger than ever before that spring. Training was smooth and unforced, despite the tremendous workload he was putting in. He recalled being in an almost perpetual state of flow in the weeks leading up to the race. When race morning arrived, he harbored the knowledge that it might just be his day.

From the start, Burfoot made himself a contender as he tucked into the front pack, comprised of a Finnish runner, several Mexican athletes, and a handful of Americans. "I recall the day very well because it was so magical," he told me in 2019. "I ran light as a feather, smooth as a steady tailwind. I recall putting almost literally no effort into the first 13 miles (21 km), even though I was with the lead group of about eight to ten."

He took stock of his feet, his breathing, and his stride. He felt a rare brush with perfection in that moment. He started to truly believe that winning might be a possibility. Then, at mile 14

(22.5 km), he told me, "I surged just a bit, just for fun. Everyone dropped back except Bill Clark."

His hopes were temporarily thwarted as he crested Heartbreak Hill with Clark still on his tail. The pair headed downhill past Boston College and toward the Evergreen Cemetery. He braced himself, waiting for Clark to come zipping by him. But then something unexpected happened: Clark's shadow disappeared. Burfoot pushed forward despite his wasted legs, entering the most populated section of the course that leads into the finish. With no barriers or crowd control, fans filled the streets, only allowing a small path for him to continue on and obstructing his view of any ensuing competition.

Sporting black shorts, a white singlet, and a white Pittsburgh Paints cap, Burfoot ran the last 100 yards (91 meters) in front of the Prudential Center, still unsure of his lead. He came across the line in first, winning in a time of 2:22:17. Clark, who had succumbed to cramping after Heartbreak Hill, crossed the finish line 32 seconds later.

In reminiscing about that day in 1968, Burfoot told me: "I honestly have never been able to understand and analyze precisely why everything came together at just the right time. I think flow is like that. I don't think you can build it with 1-2-3 instructions or simple concrete blocks. If it were that easy, we'd all have perfect race days all the time."

Harnessing a mindful mindset, identifying purpose in training, and selecting strategic goals all contribute to perfect running experiences, but as Burfoot's story illustrates, none of them matter without regular training, commitment, and practice. While the previous chapters on presence, purpose, and planning are all important to cultivating perfect running experiences, a process-focused mindset is also key. This chapter is all about how to establish a routine and approach running with a mind of intentionality.

* * *

Practice Makes Perfect

Even the early literature on the state that I classify as the perfect running experience suggests that one of the most important qualities a runner must cultivate is a certain "sticktoitiveness." This is defined by an ability to continue training even when it gets uncomfortable or frustrating, harboring faith that, over time, the training put in today will potentially make way for glimpses of perfection tomorrow.

Day-in and day-out training strengthens muscles, increases the stroke volume of your heart, builds capillaries in the muscles, increases mitochondria to produce energy, and boosts red blood cells in the bloodstream. In turn, VO2 max increases, running economy improves, and you become faster and more powerful and efficient, not to mention more resistant to fatigue. The distress signals that your heart and muscles transmit to your brain when you're out of shape dampen. What once was challenging begins to feel easier because your fitness has increased and your body is under less strain. These factors all serve to enhance your development as a runner, which feeds enjoyment of training and racing. When your body is adequately prepared for the challenge, you set yourself up for perfect running.

What runners say

A number of the runners I interviewed identified consistent training and established fitness as important to getting into that perfect running experience. Here's what some of them said:

"I think it's a matter of having dedicated time set aside for a run. Then I have nothing else to worry about because I've planned to do this race, or drive to the foothills for a trail run, or set aside a Saturday morning for a long run. That run is getting my undivided attention and that's when I think I really start to flow."

Meg S., 29, Denver, CO

"I never had any 'in the zone' runs really until I had done quite a bit of training and gained the confidence that I was a 'runner.' I think the more you train, the more confident you get that you can do it, the more flow state runs you encounter, and the more you can know what helps you have them."

Sarah E., 49, Hereford, UK

"Preparation and routine are key. Routine helps trigger a certain state, like muscle memory. Preparation removes obstacles you might stumble over—a regular running schedule, a good warm-up routine, time scheduled. It's all about consistency. Find what works, make good habits, stick with them."

Sean M., 56, Woodbridge, CT

"A lack of fitness or being very fatigued from overtraining or lack of sleep can definitely prevent one from getting in the zone."

Tom D., 58, Sydney, Australia

"Having a consistent training schedule of 30-plus miles (48 km) weekly and at least one speed work session per week is important for me to get into that headspace."

Anna D., 35, Miami, FL

"Being in great shape is a trigger for me—I don't think you can get in flow when you're struggling with basic fitness."

Jason F., 35, Denver, CO

Possibly even more important than the physical adaptations that come with regular training are the mental ones. Making running a part of your routine decreases the mental energy demands of the task of running, allowing your runs to become semi-automatic, so they are governed by less specialized and energy-zapping areas of the central nervous system. This doesn't mean that running becomes mindless, but rather, once you've trained consistently over many miles, certain things become instinctive. No matter your pace or competitive level, you no longer need to scrutinize form or constantly gauge pace, your body just knows what to do, allowing you to become totally absorbed in the whole of the experience.

The Magic of Planning Ahead: Penciling in a time to run each day takes the guesswork out of training and helps you avoid burning valuable mental energy trying to motivate yourself to squeeze in a workout. For most runners, planning workouts in one-week chunks can be a good way to stay on track. Pick a day each week to sit down and look at your schedule to figure out when and where you'll be able to fit in a run each day. If there's a day you're booked with meetings, maybe that should be an off-day. Or if there's a day you know you'll be at your child's soccer tournament from morning to night, you could consider scheduling a run from the pitches. By planning ahead, you reduce the chances of skipping workouts.

* * *

Sticking to Your Training Plan

Evolutionarily speaking, our brains are always looking for ways to conserve energy and avoid expending unnecessary effort. This frees up the mental capacity, for instance, to focus on the run itself, rather than getting bogged down trying to simply motivate yourself to run. Indeed, social psychologist Roy F. Baumeister referenced this process, coining the term "decision fatigue." This idea posits that we only have so much energy to lend to self-control. At a certain point, willpower collapses, along with focus and motivation. Selecting a training plan that fits your goals and intentions and presents an apt challenge goes a long way toward laying the groundwork for consistent running. The next challenge is to actually stick to that plan. Turning running into a habit—a predictable part of your routine—short-circuits that energy-zapping process of decision-making. By making the initial investment of consistent training, you are more likely to reap the rewards of perfect running.

Making Runs Sacred: When you're busy, running is often the first thing to get nixed from the priority list. Reframing your runs as more than just a workout or "me time" in both your own mind and the minds of your family members can help keep it from being bumped off the daily docket. Of course, unforeseen circumstances like a child's illness or family emergency might necessitate skipping a run, but other less important things won't always take the place of a workout if you've elevated the importance of running in your life. Rather than being dependent on whether you happen to have extra time to run on any given day, try making it a top priority as you work to cultivate a consistent running routine.

Fortunately, researchers believe that willpower is like a muscle—so the more consistent you are with your training, the stronger your resolve to continue to train becomes. Studies suggest that it can take anywhere from 18 days to 254 days of executing a particular task to become an ingrained habit. One of the most convincing studies concluded a middle ground of 66 days. While occasional missed workouts and inconsistencies won't serve to derail habit formation, it's important to stick with regular running as much as possible—whether that be three days a week or six—for at least a couple of months to reach that point of consistent training.

Exercise 6.1: Running Prompts

Strategically creating training prompts can help get you out the door for a run each day. Here are some examples:

- In the evening, put your running clothes in a place you will see them right away in the morning.
- Post your training plan on your refrigerator so it's one of the first things you see each morning.
- Schedule a reminder on your calendar that you're meeting a running buddy for a workout.
- Set your running shoes at the front door to serve as a reminder as soon as you get home from work.
- Put an energy bar next to your computer to signal the need for a quick snack before a lunchtime run.

One technique that can help you commit to a regular running routine is something called "scenario planning." This approach reveals how actions in the moment might potentially play out over the long haul and can be helpful to runners regardless of whether you have competitive ambitions or are running to maintain health and fitness. Large organizations often use scenario planning to make decisions about the future. In the case of a runner struggling to get out the door for regular workouts, it's worth taking a moment

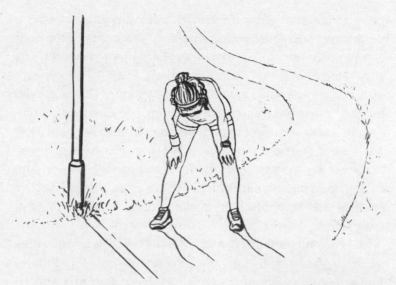

Elevating running on your priority list aids consistency in training.

to consider two possible scenarios that could occur, depending on the decisions you make after finishing work for the day:

Scenario 1

Upon returning home, you grab a snack from the kitchen and immediately collapse on the couch. It's been a long day and you're tired. You think about going for a run per your training plan later that evening. You go back and forth endlessly. Eventually, you completely lose motivation to run, so you decide to order a pizza and skip your run that day. You go to bed feeling full and uncomfortable and you wake up feeling guilty for missing another day of running.

Scenario 2

Upon returning home at the end of your work day, you grab a small snack and immediately change into your running clothes.

You're a little worn out from the day, but avoid sitting down for fear that you might lose your motivation. You head out the door for a run according to your training plan. After a successful few miles, you return home feeling energized. Instead of ordering a pizza, you are motivated to make a healthy dinner. That night you sleep better than usual and wake up feeling refreshed the next day.

While it may seem like overkill to analyze ahead of time how certain small decisions might be linked to specific consequences, it's a great way to snap yourself out of automatic pilot and into making more intentional choices. What's more, this perspective can help fuel motivation to make choices that benefit your future self.

This is why mindfulness is such a key skill—it aids in cultivating healthy habits in deliberate and intentional ways. Mindfulness allows you to co-opt the natural tendency toward mindless reactions by training your brain to examine actions in real time. As we've learned from the idea of the growth mindset, when we believe that traits and talents are not fixed and that we will reap future rewards by putting effort in today, we are far more likely to forgo the pull of chasing immediate satisfaction.

Best of all, research demonstrates that exercise is a foundational habit—one that has the power to influence a chain reaction of change in your life. For example, as you start running consistently several days a week, you might find that other healthy patterns emerge. Maybe you begin eating better and going to sleep earlier. This can signal a tectonic shift in your daily routine, having far-reaching positive implications for the landscape of your life.

Exercise 6.2: Pre-Race Routine: Applying the Art of Habit Formation to Racing

In the same way that establishing a regular running routine can take the decision fatigue out of daily training, a purposefully practiced pre-race routine can do the same for race day. A series of planned actions prior to a race can help a runner tune out distractions and focus on the task at hand. Indeed, when surveyed, competitive athletes identify a pre-competitive plan as one of the most significant factors that facilitates flow.

Dr. Cindra Kamphoff, a high-performance coach and sports psychology consultant, as well as the author of *Beyond Grit*, once told me this: "Total absorption in the task at hand allows us to more likely experience flow and reach peak performance. Performance requires us to be totally present in the here and now—if we aren't, we won't be at our best."

A pre-race routine includes everything from nutrition to warm-up. By eating the same meal, listening to the same music, and packing your race morning bag the same way, you eliminate stress and anxiety come race day.

Pre-Race Routine Components

The night before race morning:

- Gear-check: Put out your race kit to make sure everything is accounted for. Pin your race number on to your shirt and affix your timing chip to your shoe.
- Review your race plan: Take a moment to jot down your race plan step by step. This might include pace, when you'll take in nutrition, and whether or not you're planning to pick up speed later in the race. If you have mental mantras you plan on deploying at certain points during the race, log those too.
- Fuel: Eat a meal that you know will give you energy and agree with your stomach. There's no need to eat more than usual, just stick to what you know works. Also, continue to drink water and/or a sports drink, especially if you anticipate that race day weather will be hot.
- Go to sleep: Go to bed at a reasonable time, but don't worry about getting to bed extra early. Sleep the night before a race

is often fitful, so you don't want to hit the hay so early that you end up wide awake for hours cycling nervous energy.

Race morning:

- Visualize: When you wake up, spend a few moments visualizing your race and what you hope to accomplish that day. Remind yourself of any practiced mantras and try to keep your attitude trending toward positive.
- Fuel: Eat a breakfast you know works for you. Don't stuff yourself, but also make sure you get adequate calories to carry you into the race.
- Warm-up: Once you arrive at the race, do a short warm-up to loosen up your legs. Complete any special stretches or drills you usually do.

Once you've established a routine, it's important to rehearse it until it feels second nature. The best time to practice this is prior to big workouts or less important races you're doing in preparation for a big goal race. By practicing before multiple workouts and races, you'll have a good sampling of how your routine might need to be adjusted depending on things that are out of your control, like weather. With practice, this routine will go a long way towards eliminating those pre-race jitters as you toe the starting line.

***

Purposeful Practice

While subscribing to a regular training regimen and following it precisely boosts your chances of encountering more perfect running experiences, you must also remain intentional about your workouts. If you take habitual to the extreme, you risk stagnating or burning out. Research backs up this contention, finding that purposely getting out of your comfort zone lights up the learning centers of the brain and helps boost performance. It's not simply about going through the motions, but rather, keeping tabs on your goals and intentions and taking a calculated approach to each and every workout, building on lessons learned along the way. Amby Burfoot told me:

> *"I think you have to experiment — to gamble a little — to open the door that leads to perfect flow. I did some crazy stuff in training in 1968. If I hadn't, maybe I wouldn't have gotten there. I wouldn't recommend that anyone repeat my workouts, but I would suggest runners and other athletes should be willing to explore new pathways. It's so easy to get stuck in a rut; it's so hard to adventure out. But if you don't try different things, you don't learn much, and you have little chance to discover your own perfect-flow race."*

Consider the case of Paavo Nurmi, the superstar runner of the 1920s known as the "Flying Finn." He broke 22 world records in distances between 1,500 meters (1,640 yards) and 12.5 miles (20 km) and won 12 Olympic medals (nine gold) during his career. He captured the attention of Americans on his 1925 whirlwind tour of the United States during which he traveled the country competing in 55 events, 51 of which he won.

What made him so good? A pioneer when it came to training, he eschewed traditional practices and worked to develop his own techniques that allowed him to make incremental improvements. Some of these approaches continue to be used today: Year-round training that includes long-distance and speed intervals and the use of a stopwatch to ensure pacing strategy. He also reportedly employed other inventive methods that raised eyebrows—such as early forms of strength training and form drills that involved running in heavy military boots.

Rather than blindly following the accepted standard approach to training at the time, he deliberately sought out novel methods that ended up making him virtually unbeatable. Indeed, research shows that the continual practice of a skill, like running, allows us to gain a certain level of mastery, but once we get good enough for the actions to be automatic, progress levels out. For instance, when you start a training program, the body adapts by growing new capillaries to bring a greater amount of oxygen to the muscle cells in the legs, thereby making a pace that originally felt challenging rather easy. If you continue doing the exact same training, though, the development will cease and you'll remain at the same level. You must stress the body and push it to adapt if you hope to find a new homeostasis.

To continue to make improvements, we have to be purposeful about challenging ourselves, much in the manner of Nurmi. This is something Swedish psychologist Anders Ericsson calls "deliberate practice." Deliberate or purposeful practice is all about approaching each run with a specific goal and monitoring the process. Instead of mindlessly running through a workout, it's important to be deliberate about your thinking and actions if you hope to maximize potential and continue cultivating the right conditions for the perfect running experience.

Purposeful practice can mean many things to a runner and it doesn't require you to stomp out your mileage in military boots the way Nurmi did. Maybe each week you challenge yourself to add another mile on to your longest run, add an extra interval to your speed workout, or employ a new strength-training program. If health and fitness is your primary goal, maybe you up the ante by adding an extra cross-training activity to your weekly workout calendar. A more purposeful path is largely about pushing back on the tendency to fall into a fixed mindset in which you assume that you have a certain amount of innate potential, but that's as far as growth and development will go. That tactic is not designed to challenge homeostasis and help you continue to make improvements. A more deliberate approach will.

The Power of Community: The importance of taking a deliberate approach to training doesn't stop when you shed your running shoes. Intentionally surrounding yourself with people who support your training can help keep you motivated. Whether it's a spouse who serves as an energetic cheerleader from the sidelines or a training partner who holds you accountable for runs a couple days a week, having people in your life who understand and support your running is vital. There's even research to suggest that anywhere from 40 to 70 percent of your fitness level may be explained by those you surround yourself with—both good and poor fitness appears to be contagious. Don't go it alone—seek out community to help keep you on track toward achieving your running goals.

---

* * *

Monitoring the Process

Part of purposeful practice is mindfully keeping tabs on how your body and mind are progressing throughout the course of training. Ben Rosario, the coach of a group of professional runners in Flagstaff, Arizona, known as Northern Arizona Elite, told me this: "You need to be able to learn to read your internal rhythms on the fly—that comes with experience. You learn how the body feels running at certain paces and effort levels. In order to have a great race, you really have to just go by feel." There are countless tools on the market that can help you get a better handle on how your body is functioning during a run: GPS watches, heart-rate monitors, and power meters, to name a few. The latest devices can also assist in monitoring sleep and recovery. While these offer useful data on the road to more perfect running experiences, I am a proponent of learning to hone a heightened ability to listen to the body's feedback without too much reliance on external devices.

Every time you set out for a run, your body offers up information. Physical sensations, breathing rate, perceived effort, and mental clarity are all indicators of how a run is going. Think of them as the gauges on your car's dashboard display. How's your fuel supply? What about tire pressure? How about speed? What about the tachometer and oil? When you're driving, you learn to almost subconsciously pay attention to these things without over-monitoring them. You still have to keep your eyes on the road, after all.

You want to learn to do the same thing when you're running— always staying tuned in to your physical sensations enough to know if something is going awry. Many coaches refer to this as "running by feel." In the same way you wouldn't ignore a speedometer that shows you're going 20 miles an hour over the speed limit or a fuel gauge that indicates you're on an empty tank, so too should you be aware of what is going on with your body on a run in order to respond appropriately and put out small fires before they turn into raging infernos.

If you're wary of trusting your own perceptions of exertion over a power meter or heart-rate monitor, consider this: New research found that "rate of perceived exertion" or RPE was just as accurate at measuring how hard experienced athletes worked when compared to fancy technology and data analysis. Those internal metrics help you monitor your progress by offering the gift of keen insight into the inner machinations of body and brain.

We often miss vital physical clues when we are constantly distracted on a run, lost in thought, or overly focused on goals far in the future. As was discussed in Chapter 3, research suggests that leveraging the power of mindfulness is perhaps the best way to run by feel because it trains you to monitor what's happening in the present moment. Dr. Rick Hecht, a professor of medicine and the research director at the Osher Center for Integrative Medicine at the University of California, San Francisco, as well as a seasoned ultrarunner, told me this: "Mindfulness can help you discriminate the difference between the discomfort associated with a hard effort in training or racing and one that is going to lead to injury. From my personal experience, it helps me pay attention to my body's cues and signals when I'm running."

Doing a mindful head-to-toe body scan, as described in Chapter 3, is a great way to dial in to your physical senses. The observations you make during these scans gives you a read on how your body is feeling overall. While you can't assume you need a day off of training at the first sign of fatigue or discomfort—that's part of the training process, after all—gaining an ardent awareness of how your body is operating on the run assists you in identifying when something is amiss or, conversely, when you can push harder toward a breakthrough. It's about learning to let your body guide training, not just what you have written on your training calendar.

Exercise 6.3: Mindfully Examining Pain and Discomfort on the Run

While practicing mindfulness will help build a natural sense of body awareness to clue you in when something is going haywire, here are a few questions to ask yourself if you experience any pain or discomfort on a run. Your answers will help you determine if the sensations are associated with the inherent discomfort of running or an impending injury, which will guide you to keep pushing or back off.

- Have I felt this pain before?
- Could this be related to a past injury?
- Is it a shooting, sharp pain or a dull ache?
- Is my current mood influencing how my body feels?

Exercise 6.4: Your Hourglass of Energy

Learning to listen to your body can help you avoid injuries and overtraining. It can also help you put in more productive and enjoyable mileage by teaching you how to monitor energy expenditure. I envision the runner's body like an "energy hourglass." As you push in a workout or race, for instance, grains of sand fall through the hourglass from top to bottom. The harder or longer you push, the faster the sand falls. Once all of the sand is at the bottom of the hourglass, your energy stores are depleted. To keep your energy stores in check and make sure you don't let all the sand slip through the hourglass before the end of a workout or the finish of a race, remember the following acronym and ask yourself these questions:

S: Starting point—How do I feel both physically and mentally prior to today's run?

A: Attitude—How am I feeling overall about the run today? Are my thoughts more positive or negative? Am I feeling healthy, sick, well rested, or stressed?

N: Needs—What other responsibilities and commitments do I have today that require energy?

D: Distance—How many miles do I have planned? Does this feel achievable today?

S: Speed—What is my prescribed pacing plan? Does it feel hard or easy today?

While putting in hard work to boost fitness is vital, rigidly sticking to a training plan and grinding through workouts that your body and mind are resisting is counterproductive. Learning to keep tabs on the intensity level of your exercise is a key aspect of running by feel. Your rate of perceived exertion on a run will tell you whether you're working too hard or not hard enough. It offers a general

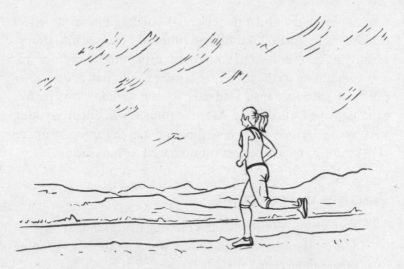

A purposeful approach to training can help you discover more perfect runs.

sense of how you are feeling, taking into account things like heart rate, breathing, and muscle fatigue. Here is a quick reference to keep in mind as you run.

Respiration: Is your breathing shallow, deep, quick, relaxed, rhythmic, or erratic?

Muscles: Does your body feel heavy or light? Is your leg turnover fast or strained? Do you feel tense or relaxed?

Mind: Are you focused or distracted?

Attitude: Are you feeling more positive or negative about the run? Are you enjoying yourself or hating every minute of it?

Thinking about these things can help capture how you're feeling overall. Not only can learning to listen to your body in this way boost performance, it also increases the likelihood of finding your way into that perfect running state.

So far, we've examined the essential building blocks to perfect running experiences: Establishing mindful presence in training, identifying purpose behind your running, planning a way forward, and committing to the process. Chapter 7 will look at one other potential path that may lead you toward entering that perfect running state: Participation. As some runners will discover, taking what you've learned so far and applying it to the group, team, or club setting can make perfect running well within reach.

Practices in Perfection

- A commitment to consistent training has important physical and psychological implications when it comes to priming that optimal state.
- Making running a regular part of your routine helps breed motivation in training.
- A commitment to process over end goals is essential to discovering more perfect runs.
- Purposeful practice helps you stay on track with your goals and intentions for running.
- Learning to mindfully listen to your body throughout training is essential to healthy and successful running and performance.

CHAPTER 7
PARTICIPATION

"Whether it's just two runners doing a workout together, a team workout of 30–100 people, or a marathon with 30,000 runners, group settings offer the opportunity to feed off of each other's energy. The back-and-forth that can happen produces a mutual sense of purpose and euphoria. There's something really synergistic about it."

IN LATE JANUARY, just three weeks before the 2016 U.S. Olympic Marathon Trials were to be held in Los Angeles, three elite marathoners from the Northern Arizona Elite team set out for their last big workout. The group, which is based in Flagstaff, is home to some of the best runners in the country. Among the team preparing for the trials was 2:12-marathoner Matt Llano, 2:14-marathoner Scott Smith, and 2:24-marathoner Kellyn Taylor.

During their 12-week buildup to the big race, the team met daily for runs, as well as for strength and conditioning work. While there are a number of professional training groups around the country, NAZ Elite is known for being particularly tight-knit. This is by design—positive team chemistry is a must, according to head coach Ben Rosario, a 2:18-marathoner and former professional runner himself. Establishing the group's home base in Flagstaff was also purposeful. A running mecca of sorts, it sits at 7,000 feet (2,134 meters) and is noted for its extensive trail system and wide variety of terrain.

The day before their last high-pressure workout leading up to the trials, the group packed up their cars and made the four-hour drive to Lake Mead, just outside of Las Vegas. They sought out this lower altitude locale in hopes of simulating the course they would encounter in Los Angeles. Upon arrival, Rosario hauled out his measuring wheel and walked a four-mile out-and-back course, marking every quarter mile to help his athletes stay on pace throughout the workout.

Intimidated by the difficulty of the course, Taylor remembered, "When we arrived at Lake Mead the day before the workout, our initial reaction was less than positive. We knew that it was going to be a really difficult workout to hit."

"We didn't really have any other option but to attack this thing without too much reservation" added Smith. "I think we got all our apprehension out the night before when we got to jog the course Ben laid out. There is a big difference between jogging a course and trying to run it at race pace though. I was certainly nervous, but more so I was at peace with whatever was going to happen that day. There was definitely a feeling of delving into the unknown, which is great practice for racing."

The next morning, Llano, Smith, and Taylor arrived ready to take on the 16-mile (25.75-km) tempo run at marathon pace on that four-mile course. The plan was for Smith to run 4:57 mile pace, Llano to run 4:59 pace, and Taylor to run 5:35 pace. The week before, their teammate Ben Bruce, who was also preparing for the marathon trials, ran a personal best half marathon of 1:02:28. This boosted the spirits of not only Bruce, but also his teammates who had been training with him.

"My favorite part about the marathon trials segment of training was getting to do the work with a big group," said Taylor. "We weren't running the same paces, but just knowing that we were all out there suffering for the same goal was special. It provided a sense of accountability and calm."

The three runners warmed up together and completed mobility drills in an old parking lot. The mood was punctuated by a nervous energy. All knew that a good result in this workout boded well for their chances at the trials. Smith recalled:

"The beginning of the workout felt a little daunting. I just remember starting downhill heading straight toward Lake Mead at the crack of dawn. It was almost a bit eerie, but it was also exciting. This was an entirely new training venue for us and I don't think any of us had a firm grasp on the best way to run the route Ben designed. There were a lot of turns and some uphill and downhill miles so we definitely were aware that we would not be running even splits. I remember having kind of a business trip mentality, which I think was shared by Matt and Kellyn. We were here to do a job and we were going to do it to the best of our abilities. I think we brought that mindset to almost every workout that segment and it was really an exciting time for the team."

From the moment Rosario and his athletes punched the start buttons on their watches, it became clear that something special was coming together after months of training. "I vividly remember that workout. The vibe among those athletes was really good. I loved the atmosphere. It's hard to explain, but an athlete just gets this tingle in their body where they feel like it's just going to go well from the start," Rosario told me.

As the runners clicked off each two-mile stretch, he recalls a fluidity in their execution. Even when they weren't running side by side, they appeared to feed off of one another's energy. "As a coach, I watched them cruise along, so locked into what they were doing. There was no negativity and a total fearlessness in the way they were approaching this session together," he added. "They were really in sync and invested in the workout together in a way that was very cool."

"I remember starting to flow, I don't really know if it was necessarily in some sort of metaphysical sense, but I'm a pretty good downhill runner and just started letting it roll. I stopped worrying about splits and just let go," said Smith. "I definitely was leaning into the effort and it was one of the few times in my running career where it seemed like there was no bottom to the well. Every time I pushed there was more. That is a fun place to be in a workout or race and I try to remember and cherish those moments because they are pretty rare for me."

As they rounded into the final mile and crossed the proverbial finish line, they each clicked their watches. Taylor recalled: "We all hit our prescribed paces. We had successfully finished the biggest workout of the segment. We were ready." Smith said it was a turning point in his training for the trials. "It was like getting in a car without having any idea how many gears it has," he recalled. "You start redlining one gear and decide to see if there's another, and another, and another. It felt like that day there was no end to the gears. It was by far the best workout I had done to that point in my career."

While some runners prefer to train alone, running in the company of others can invoke powerful experiences and elevated performances. As the NAZ Elite runners can attest, a special kind of perfect running experience can arise when you're in pursuit of a common objective with other runners. This chapter is all about how "group flow" can offer yet another avenue into that perfect running state.

* * *

Group Flow

Running is widely considered a solo sport. Alan Sillitoe's landmark story published in 1959, "The Loneliness of the Long-Distance Runner," is oft-referenced in running circles and beyond, further cementing the image of running as a solitary pursuit. In the story, Sillitoe's lonely hero, Colin Smith, identifies running as a venue through which he is able to experience the world in solitude. For many high school, college, elite, and adult teams and clubs, however, running is a highly social activity. Indeed, as the workout executed by the NAZ Elite team demonstrates, it may even create an environment that is more conducive to perfect running experiences than running on your own.

"If you're having trouble reaching flow on your own because your mind isn't in the right place—maybe you're too focused on the negative or not excited about the challenge—training in a group can be a great thing," elite coach and exercise physiologist Greg McMillan told me. "It might help you develop better focus and be more open to the experience of pushing yourself, which can increase that probability of reaching that flow state."

Head coach of New York City's Central Park Track Club and member of the 1980 Puerto Rican Olympic team, Tony Ruiz, echoed those sentiments when he told me, "Whether it's just two runners doing a workout together, a team workout of 30–100 people, or a marathon with 30,000 runners, group settings offer the opportunity to feed off of each other's energy. The back-and-forth that can happen produces a mutual sense of purpose and euphoria. There's something really synergistic about it."

In fact, research has shown that social flow experiences are often identified as more enjoyable than solitary flow experiences. In cultural anthropology, this might be dubbed "collective effervescence" or "communitas"—the deep and evocative

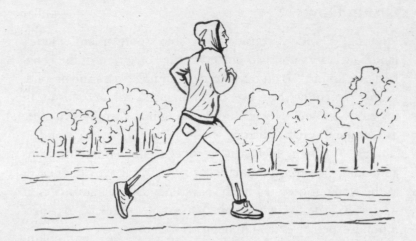

Some runners will find that flow is more easily reached in the group setting.

feelings of belonging and oneness that result from richly meaningful and transcendent shared experiences. Group flow is also sometimes referred to as "relational flow," "shared flow," "co-flow," and "team flow." While Csikszentmihalyi's research largely focuses on individual flow experiences, the literature also chronicles surgeons reporting the sensation of an entire surgical team operating as a single organism, jazz musicians playing spontaneously in tandem, and even the dynamics between members of a Japanese motorcycle gang.

While the research on group flow is still emerging, one of the fields it is most commonly referenced in is the sporting world. As it turns out, although running is largely thought of as a solo endeavor, its rhythmic nature and the fact that it generally involves all members of the team executing the same action together— even at different paces—make it a particularly apt sport through which to achieve the team flow experience.

A number of the coaches I talked to explained how shared suffering on a run also naturally brings athletes together. "I've witnessed group flow a lot, especially when I coached the McMillan Elite Team," McMillan told me. "It gives runners purpose—that shared experience of suffering together and celebrating in each other's successes. It's this mutual understanding that even though you are competing individually, you're all running together and lifting each other up. When one runner is having a good day, there is a snowball effect for their teammates."

Luke Humphrey, a two-time Olympic Marathon Trials qualifier and former member of the professional Hansons-Brooks Original Distance Project based in Rochester, Michigan, said this: "What would have been a daunting workout was made possible by training together as a group. We all took turns sharing the workload of setting the pace so we'd be thinking about that responsibility to the team and getting the guys through our next mile, not so much the pace itself. Then the pace would just take care of itself. There really was comfort in suffering through a workout with teammates—a true sense of camaraderie."

Ben Rosario shared this of the NAZ elite runners: "Only they could possibly know how much they were suffering. Sharing that suffering is a unique thing and it can only happen when you're training hard with other runners. When you're training for a big important event together, the atmosphere is heightened."

Perfect running in the group setting is much like the other types of optimal experiences discussed throughout this book, but it has the potential to be more powerful because a greater number of factors must align for it to come about. When a sense of movement coalesces and collective consciousness convenes, each individual experience and performance is elevated. The Theory of Social Facilitation suggests just this—that when you execute a practiced activity in the presence of other people, performance improves. To be sure, as McMillan alludes, runners tend to run faster in team training environments than they often would on their own.

"Sometimes a team or club will have a great day and you wonder, 'why that day?'" added McMillan. "If everyone is fresh and someone is pushing the pace and the members of the group are rising to the occasion, there's this collective feeling of 'wow, we are doing great!' This allows individual runners to get more out of themselves than they normally would. You can see how momentum forms in those scenarios."

One of the most common venues where runners of all experience levels and paces encounter group flow is in road races. While you may have logged most of your training miles on your own, you often end up running with several of the same people during a race. Pace aligns and an unspoken bond forms among strangers. You may not utter a single word to one another, but somehow you feel a familiarity. You're enduring the highs and lows of running and experiencing the sights and sounds of the race together. "When you're running a marathon and you see pace groups—crowds of runners somehow all come together based on the same pace and finishing goal. There's a spontaneous bond that happens there that's really cool. It's part of why runners love the sport so much and stand around talking at the finish line forever—it's that shared experience," added McMillan.

Humphrey, now a coach and author of the popular *Hansons Marathon Method*, described experiencing a similar phenomenon among his elite teammates at the 2006 Boston Marathon. As individual athletes from the group logged impressive breakthroughs that season, the entire team began to develop a strong sense of belief in their fitness. That day at the Boston Marathon, a number of seemingly imperfect factors culminated to produce a sense of perfection.

"We were running in the biggest race in the world with guys we had literally run thousands of miles with. It calmed us down and it allowed us to be in the moment and not get overwhelmed," recalled Humphrey. "It also allowed us to dig deeper than we thought possible. The end result was amazing as we put six guys in the top 22 at a time when the American presence on the world stage was nearly absent."

This result may have been partially due to a phenomenon known as the Emotional Contagion Theory, which suggests that one person's emotions and behaviors can trigger similar emotions and behaviors among the people around them. We tend to unconsciously mirror one another. When a couple of runners in a group exude confidence and focus, others tend to pick up on that. Rosario put it this way: "In group flow there is this overall vibe where everyone is running at their best, they are hitting their times, and there's a great overall attitude among the runners."

Perfect running is no exception. Experts suggest that when conditions are right and certain members of a group enter the flow state, becoming so-called agents of flow, it can spread and become a collective social experience. This is similar to the "hive mind" concept in sociology that captures the notion of collective consciousness. When a group or even a pair of runners are in a unified pursuit of a challenging objective, strides sync, pace coalesces, and the group metaphorically morphs into something like a superorganism.

Many of the factors that contribute to perfect running in the group setting parallel those of individual flow. In the same way, all of these things don't need to be present for group flow to arise. Depending on the group make-up—a high school or college team, an adult running club, a pair of marathon training buddies, or an elite team—differences exist. Consider the following potential precursors to the perfect running experience in the group setting.

Shared goals

Common goals—long-term, short-term, and micro—among runners can help set the stage for group flow. With that said, goals will vary widely depending on the dynamics of the group. For instance, a cross-country squad may unite around the long-term goal of winning a state title and a small group of running buddies might decide to work to set personal bests in an end-of-season 5k race. "Similar mindsets form especially when communication is good among a group of runners training together," McMillan explained. "They might all think, 'We are going to do something great, this is our year!'" Shared objectives may be enough to induce that perfect running experience during group workouts, which are designed to build toward that long-term goal. Rosario offered similar sentiments:

> "Part of the groundwork is laid over time as you train together and some of it can be created in a more formal way in team meetings when you all get together and say, "Hey, this is what we are doing." There's a certain bravery involved in saying "Let's do this" in front of others – it's important to experience that vulnerability together. It's about deciding that as a group you're going to work really hard to try to do something special – something that maybe the individual runners can't do alone, but together they are able to rise to the occasion."

Short-term goals can also contribute to group flow. These may include finishing a specific workout or completing a high-mileage week of training together. For newer runners, it may mean committing to meeting a running buddy several times a week to jumpstart training. Weekend long runs organized by training groups are a great example of the type of scenario where a perfect run might arise. The shared experience of pushing for a long distance can create conditions that are amenable to that perfect running state.

Micro goals are another common trigger. Maybe you're out for a moderately paced run with a 5K training group and one runner suggests picking up the pace for a mile or adding on a bit of extra distance. When the group is comprised of like-minded individuals with similar motivations, these spontaneous objectives are embraced by the group. On teams that harbor undue pressure on athletes to perform, tweaks to training often diminish the running experience for many of the group's members. A more cohesive unit will make decisions on the fly and embrace a flow-inducing spirit of shared improvement.

Exercise 7.1: Group Goal Setting

Research has demonstrated that the process of discussing and refining goals can play an integral role in a team's unity and raison d'être. Since runners will have their own objectives, personal goals and group goals must be compatible. When goal setting is done in a collaborative way, individuals adopt the team goals as part of their personal mission.

In the same way I recommend in Chapter 5 that individual runners choose S.M.A.R.T. goals (Specific, Measurable, Achievable, Relevant, Time-Bound), so too should teams. Before defining group goals, each runner should already have established personal goals for the season. Then athletes can begin to reflect on their hopes for the team and how that fits with their individual goals. Each member of the group should contribute ideas. Input should be logged in order to identify patterns and encourage discussion. While clubs and teams might organize a goal-setting session where everyone chimes in regarding their ambitions for the group, running buddies or smaller groups could utilize a less formal method of establishing objectives.

When all is said and done, you should be able to settle on at least one big goal for the group and several secondary goals. A college team may set their sights on a regional title and a marathon training group may resolve to get everyone to the starting line of a goal race healthy and fit. Similarly, a pair of running buddies might set a goal of meeting twice a week to train together and a beginning running group could work to make sure every member finishes a 5K. Goals can look very different depending on the group, but all of these objectives contribute to creating a successful team atmosphere that fosters many chances for perfect running.

Shared purpose

A holistic focus develops when athletes feel they are part of a shared mission. Coach Tony Ruiz told me this: "A shared sense of purpose is vital. As a coach of a sizeable group, it's my job to set up workouts that benefit everyone. I always explain how the workout is designed and what the goal is so that every runner understands why they are doing what they are doing."

This phenomenon is characterized by a meaningful understanding of the self as part of a larger whole. This means that each runner must align their thoughts and actions with the objectives of the team at large. To do this, individual runners focus on their personal contributions, while remaining keenly aware of the common purpose. The same distinction that exists between goals and purpose for individuals also exists for groups. While a club or team may have a concrete long-term goal, their mission statement should be concerned with the group's purpose, beliefs about how the team should operate, and team values.

Exercise 7.2: Developing a Team Mission Statement

A team mission statement should be clear, concise, and inspirational. Research suggests that answering the following three questions can be helpful in developing a group mission statement:

1. Who are we as a team?
2. What do we hope to do this season and in the future?
3. What steps do we need to take to travel that journey?

Work with the other runners in the group to answer these questions and form a one-sentence mission statement. Here are a couple of examples:

"The club seeks to provide a supportive atmosphere where runners of all skill levels and backgrounds are offered the chance to experience the joy of running."

"The team will foster growth and development by providing runners with opportunities to learn and train in a safe, equitable, and fun environment."

Shared focus and engagement

Experts suggest that to achieve a shared state of optimal experience, each member of the group must be completely absorbed in the activity. This goes hand in hand with cultivating a mindful approach to training and racing. When each runner works to be fully present, they are more likely to become immersed in the experience and fall into sync with other runners around them.

Getting everyone to be on the same page in the moment can be tricky and usually only comes with practice. When it does occur, runners are able to adjust pace or tactical moves on the fly with little to no communication. This happens because everyone is so dialed in to that moment, they intuitively respond together. It's all about eschewing distractions that interfere with executing the task at hand and training each individual runner to mindfully approach training and racing.

Exercise 7.3: Mindful Walking

Before you can run, you must learn to walk. To help cultivate the perfect running experience among a group of runners, work on honing present-moment awareness together via this mindful walking exercise. You'll find that it can help you begin to direct a spirit of mindfulness toward physical movement. Once you master this, you should be able to apply it to runs. Follow these steps:

1. Find a quiet spot large enough for everyone to walk 11–16 yards (10–15 meters).
2. Instruct athletes to do the following:

   a. Focus on the moment by closing your eyes, standing in a relaxed pose, and taking three slow, deep breaths.

   b. Open your eyes and begin to slowly walk in a straight line.

   c. Notice how it feels to pick your foot up off the ground, deliberately swing your leg forward, and plant your foot.

   d. Pay attention to each movement and the associated sensations.

   e. If you get distracted, simply notice that you've lost focus and redirect to your feet.

   f. Continue walking back and forth for five minutes. Try to stay in the moment as much of that time as possible.

   g. When the time is up, take a few moments to discuss the exercise among the group. Was it hard or easy to stay focused? Did anything surprise you? How might you carry over this present-moment concentration to group runs?

Team chemistry

While we don't always have the opportunity to hand-select the runners we train with in group and team settings, chemistry often arises spontaneously. Consider those who join a running club to prepare for a marathon—many will naturally be like-minded and share similar goals. The same goes for beginner running groups. When personalities peacefully merge, this sets the stage for those perfect group runs.

That's exactly what Ruiz has witnessed with his runners over the years. "Clubs like ours offer a unique camaraderie, like a family. You share a common goal and meet twice and sometimes three times a week to pursue it," he explained. "It's not uncommon for people on our team to run together year after year through many life stages. As a result, a really positive atmosphere and overall energy develops."

Good chemistry among runners arises from a supportive environment in which all athletes are viewed on a level playing field. While different paces and ability levels might exist, there needs to be a sense of equality and mutual support among members. As McMillan told me, "If you have a group with an outstanding athlete who feels too good for everyone else, that creates friction. It's important to have runners who compete with, not against their teammates. The way some athletes approach training has a way of getting the best out of the runners around them. When athletes are team players and understand the importance of the team effort, that mentality spreads and everyone starts to perform better."

Humphrey said that a shared sense of purpose helped to cultivate chemistry among the Hansons-Brooks athletes he ran with. "We came from all different backgrounds, but the one thing we had in common was that we all wanted to accomplish the same things and so that minimized any differences," he told me. "We also all wanted to work, listen, learn, and perform. I think the group was always blessed with teammates who were leaders, nurturers, and butt kickers in the right balance."

Exercise 7.4: Building Chemistry

While chemistry can naturally materialize, sometimes it needs a little nudge. Here are three ways to encourage chemistry to develop among a group of runners:

1. Promote a sense of belonging: When runners feel supported by their training partners, chemistry is more likely to develop. Work to foster an environment that promotes communication between athletes. Runners who know that their teammates care about how they are doing both in training and life will feel a greater bond with one another.

2. Organize social outings: Getting a group of runners together outside of the training environment can be a great way to build these bonds. Organizing a team meal or other social outing gets athletes talking about their lives outside of running, which leads to greater mutual understanding and trust between athletes.

3. Mix things up: Relationships often stagnate when members of a running club or team do the same things in training every time they meet. Scheduling a team cross-training activity or "fun run" can get athletes out of their comfort zones and may even level the playing field between runners of varying ability levels. Non-traditional training days keep things from getting too serious and help athletes loosen up around one another.

Motivational balance

Research suggests that when you believe that your performance may in some way benefit or inspire others, motivation and performance improve. "When the spirit of the group surrounds running not just for yourself, but the benefit of the team, that can positively influence motivation. It's this feeling of genuinely wanting everyone to do better," explained McMillan. A supportive bond among runners can make way for perfect running to arise.

As we've seen, the perfect running state further improves the performances of all involved.

"Running with a group can be powerful," added Humphrey. "The sense of community that it brings is unprecedented, but I think it also can show a runner how much more we are capable of than maybe we let ourselves think. Seeing a peer make a big step and knowing that you are doing the same thing that they are doing in training can be a huge motivator."

It is important to note that there is a dark side to running with a group—which is excessive pressure to perform. If a runner doesn't feel full autonomy and is pushed to perform, tension arises. For perfect running to be accessible, there needs to be an understanding that everyone will run to the best of their abilities on that day. Period. When things don't go according to plan, it is vital that teammates still support each other in order not to jeopardize long-term bonds.

Exercise 7.5: Group Training for Varying Skill and Experience Levels

When runners within a group are at differing fitness or ability levels, it can be difficult to figure out how to offer that balance between skill and challenge that is necessary to create perfect running experiences. As we've discussed, when there is a mismatch between the runner's skill set and the difficulty of the task, anxiety or boredom arises. In either case, perfect running becomes unreachable. So how might an experienced age-group champion successfully find flow running with a newer runner who is still working to get into shape?

A number of options exist, but all involve workouts that allow runners to train in the same venue at differing paces. An interval workout on a track is the best example. In this case, the entire team might warm up and cool down together, but the main part of the workout differs depending on the athlete. While runners are executing varying numbers of intervals at a variety of paces, a spirit of "we are in this together" can still develop. What's more, since everyone is executing their workout in the same place, words of encouragement can be offered throughout. These types of environments have the potential to sow the seeds for group flow even when runners aren't technically running together for much of the workout.

Group cohesion

Group cohesion is the process in which members of a group bond and work together toward a common objective. Research demonstrates that team cohesion is vital for setting the stage for optimal experiences. "Cohesion is a requirement—it certainly was for the McMillan Elite team. It was about having the right athletes at the right time where you saw that flow happening and the team was really lifting up the individual athletes' performances," McMillan told me.

There are a number of factors that can help establish cohesiveness among a group of runners. First and foremost is team chemistry, as was just discussed. The Social Identity Theory demonstrates that people tend to feel closer to those with whom they think they share similarities. Even runners who come from wholly different backgrounds may discover cohesiveness via a mutual love for running or a shared goal. The social psychology literature also suggests that group size plays a role. Smaller or moderately sized teams or clubs may find it easier to establish cohesion.

Finally, group identity bolsters cohesion. Identity may arise from the prestige attached to belonging to a certain team or a record of past success. It might also be associated with long-standing team traditions or a shared commitment to the group's mission and purpose. No matter how it is formed, group identity and pride fosters a sense of unity and oneness.

Exercise 7.6: Team Trigger Words and Phrases

Developing team cohesion among runners comes naturally for some teams and clubs, but is trickier for others. While there are a number of ways to build cohesion, one of my favorites is creating cue words or motivational phrases that everyone identifies with. This positive language is designed to trigger certain actions or mental shifts.

So how might you come up with a cue word or phrase? Schedule a meeting of the minds and have runners all contribute ideas. In most cases, certain words or phrases will resonate with many of the athletes. You could decide on something as simple as "BAM!" to signal a surge in a race or "PUSH!" to deploy in the final stretch. Once you've settled on one or two, as well as added some context for what the word should signal, begin using it in workouts so it becomes a permanent part of every runner's mental arsenal.

Some other ideas:

- "Breathe"
- "Focus"
- "Fast feet"
- "Dig deep"

Collective efficacy

Collective efficacy is the team version of self-belief—it is the shared and unified belief that a group is capable of meeting certain objectives together. Put simply, there needs to be shared belief in the collective power of the group to induce co-flow. In the case of perfect group runs, this means that not only should the individuals believe in their own abilities, but they also need to feel a sense of faith in their teammates and the group at large.

"The East Africans are the best example of this," said McMillan. "In those large training groups in Kenya, hundreds of athletes train together and one runner will see another runner race really well and then think, 'I can do that.' It helps build that belief and self-confidence. A single runner in the group has the ability to raise everyone's performances up."

To be sure, in the *Journal of Psychology*, Spanish researchers confirmed that collective efficacy predicts flow in groups. This is probably partially due to the fact that a sense of shared belief can reduce the distraction of the fear of failure, thereby giving the individuals in the group a sense of control and confidence that they can safely take calculated and relevant risks—like pushing a little harder than they thought possible. It is when everyone is performing optimally that those perfect runs are most likely to materialize.

"It is so important for everybody to be on the same page and believe in what they're doing and in one another," added Rosario. "From a group perspective, if everything clicks and everyone believes in the process and is confident in themselves, the entire group feels it. That type of momentum can't be stopped."

Exercise 7.7: How to Build Self-Efficacy in Runners

Research shows that individual self-efficacy, the belief in oneself, can positively influence collective efficacy. As such, building up each runner's "can-do" attitude is essential. Here are a few ways to boost self-efficacy:

1. Celebrate small individual wins: It's important to recognize progress in training. It could be the longest run you've ever completed or a personal best time set in a mile time trial— whatever the benchmark, acknowledging these seemingly small accomplishments can help to slowly build confidence and belief in oneself.

2. Take note of other runners' accomplishments: As McMillan explained, when a runner observes a training partner accomplish something, it naturally makes them reflect on their own abilities. Maybe your running buddy logged a fast 5K or finished an extra interval in a workout and you think, "Hey, maybe I can do that too!"

3. Reflect: Taking time to reflect on your past accomplishments motivates you to pursue future goals. If you find confidence is waning, look back at your training log or spend time chatting with a training partner about what they observed you've been capable of in the past. These little reminders of the things you've already accomplished are often enough to build a strong sense of inner belief in your potential.

Positive team culture

Research out of the Netherlands demonstrates that positive affect and strong relationships among team members have a snowball effect. Dubbed the "Positive Group Affect Spiral," the researchers suggest that positive attitudes, relationships, and overall group chemistry build upon and strengthen one another. A motivational environment underscored by positive social interactions are key when it comes to creating perfect running experiences in group settings.

Indeed, a positive group culture is often responsible for fostering a love for the sport among members. As has already been discussed, intrinsic motivation is a prerequisite for perfect running experiences and it is thought that those who are intrinsically motivated are not only more likely to experience flow themselves, they also are more adept at rousing others to enter that state. Shared intrinsic motivation breeds collective ambition, enhanced performance, and optimal experience within a group.

Exercise 7.8: How to Find the Perfect Training Group

For adult runners, there are often many options when it comes to running clubs and training groups. In fact, it may be hard to know which will be the best fit for you. Here are a few key questions to ask before signing up and paying your dues:

1. What types of runners does the group primarily attract?

Pace, distance, age, and gender may all be relevant demographics to look into. In particular, you'll want to know what distance most runners in the group are training for, whether they are focused on road or trail running, how fast they are, and how much weekly mileage they run. Experience level is also important to take into account. Some groups cater to beginners, others are primarily composed of veterans, and some attract runners of all paces.

2. What is the club culture like?

Some groups are more competitive, while others are focused on more recreational running and social interactions. Consider what you're looking for and how your personality might fit into the group.

3. When and where does the group meet?

Convenience is key for most runners. If the times or workout venues are going to be hard for you to make work in your schedule, you likely won't stick with the group. Most clubs meet anywhere from one to three times a week. Find out whether they expect members to show up for regular workouts or if it's on a drop-in basis. Also, be sure meeting locations are convenient. If the group meets across town, is getting there on time after work realistic? The closer the location is to your work or home, often the better.

4. Do they provide coaching?

While most running clubs have a coach at the helm, find out their level of involvement. Will they provide individualized workouts? Can they help you plan out an entire training program? If you're simply looking for people to run with, this may not matter, but if you're hoping for some guidance, coaching is a major benefit.

5. Can you join any time?
Some groups have more structured programs that have start and end dates, while others run all year round with members training for a wide variety of races. Find out if their schedule works for your needs.

***

The Benefits of Group Flow

The collective perfect running experience tends to reinforce many of the factors that lead to the phenomenon in the first place. While positive team chemistry is a necessary prerequisite for collective flow, chemistry is bolstered by this shared experience. In the same way, group identity and motivation will enjoy a boost when a team experiences optimal experiences together. As such, bonds between teammates are elevated.

Additionally, researchers believe that collective flow improves performance in a wide range of activities, from sports, to creative endeavors, to corporate settings. In the case of a group of runners, those experiences of perfect running synchrony can prompt individual runners to redouble their efforts toward achieving both their own personal goals and the goals of the group. As Rosario told me, "When you're able to train in that heightened state with a group, everyone tends to perform at a higher level."

This can be partially attributed to a strengthened sense of intrinsic motivation to run, which is a natural by-product of the perfect running experience. Indeed, it can augment a runner's

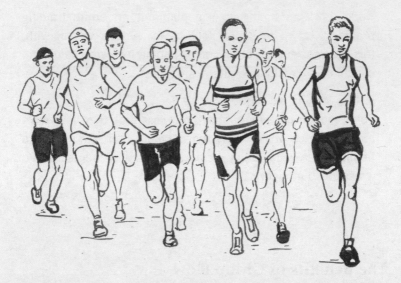

Collective flow elevates the individual runners as well as the group as a whole.

sense of meaning and purpose, which positively influences commitment, as well as individual and group performance. Rosario has experienced this phenomenon first hand, explaining to me, "It is intoxicating. Every time you feel that flow is another day that gets you more and more hooked on the sport. You want to have that feeling again. When you experience it, it inspires this internal drive to get back to that place."

Collective flow experiences also tend to enhance a runner's confidence in both themselves and the team. When team members are mutually committed to training, they share a desire to support one another. This encourages greater engagement, which naturally contributes to improved performance. Team flow is a sure sign that a group is flourishing. The synergistic nature of a perfect running experience breeds more perfect running experiences, creating a virtuous cycle. When the right runners and the right environment and training come together to produce this, every athlete's relationship with running is elevated.

Should You Join a Running Club?

Some runners prefer to go it alone, while others love the camaraderie of a running club. Here are a few of the top reasons to give group running a try:

- More perfect runs: For some runners, flow becomes more accessible in the group setting. If you are struggling to find flow, consider seeking out a training partner or group who might help you enter that unique state on the run.

- Better performance: Running with others often brings out the best in us. We are challenged to push ourselves to new speeds and distances that we may not have attempted on our own.

- Training guidance: Most clubs have at least one coach to provide expert advice to its members. From workout prescriptions to knowledge about injuries and supplemental training, a coach can play a major role in contributing to improved performance.

- Safety: There is strength in numbers. Especially if you find yourself running before or after dark or in more secluded locations, joining a running club is a great way to ensure safety.

- Novelty: For runners who are stuck in their ways, a running club can open up a whole new world—new routes, new races, new workouts, and new training partners. All of these things have the potential to inspire a renewed sense of motivation to run.

- Social bonds: One of the biggest perks of joining a running club is the fast friendships that are forged. Not only will those friends keep you accountable in training, they'll also make it a whole lot more fun.

Now that we've covered the most direct paths that lead toward the perfect running experience, we will turn our attention to some of the smaller things you can do to set the odds in your favor. Chapter 8 includes information about what type of workouts can facilitate these experiences, as well as the importance of the environment in which you choose to run. While there are no guarantees, taking these actions stacks the deck in your favor.

Practices in Perfection

- For some runners, the perfect running experience can be easier to cultivate in the company of other runners.
- Running provides a unique opportunity to experience group flow because of the rhythm of the movement and the fact that everyone is executing the same task.
- Precursors to the perfect running experience in the group setting include: Shared goals, shared purpose, shared focus and engagement, team chemistry, motivational balance, group cohesion, collective efficacy, and positive team culture.
- Group flow can improve relationships between runners, increase enjoyment of training, and boost individual and team performance.

CHAPTER 8
PUTTING THE PRINCIPLES OF PERFECT RUNNING INTO MOTION

"I just accepted the conditions and soon found myself moving with the course, rather than against it. I found lines I hadn't seen before, places to push the pace, and figured out how to navigate the headwinds and eventually I was moving. I wasn't pushing, but I was moving more and more ahead. I was just in the moment and that allowed me to release all expectations and flow."

ON JANUARY 31, 2019, 40 runners crossed under a narrow start banner on a snow- and ice-covered airfield runway on the middle of a glacier in Novo, Antarctica—known as the highest, windiest, emptiest, and coldest place on Earth. Snow squeaking and crunching underfoot, the runners cautiously navigated the rutted, amorphous terrain. The windswept landscape revealed a lonely ice desert unfolding in every direction all around them, buffered by jagged crystalline mountains in the distance.

The group, clad in goggles and parkas, looked more like the ski patrol than a group of runners. Even so, they were all there for a special event: The Antarctica Intercontinental Marathon. Part of the World Marathon Challenge, these harriers were poised to complete seven marathons on seven continents in seven consecutive days, starting in Novo.

The logistics of the annual challenge are staggering: Participants run 183 miles (294.5 km) over seven days and spend around

63 hours in the air, taking charter flights from one marathon to the next. They often sleep in cramped planes and are constantly working to adjust to jet lag. The 2019 event kicked off with runners navigating six and a half loops of the perimeter of that icy airfield runway in Novo, one they had just landed on hours earlier in a Boeing 757 VIP from Cape Town, South Africa.

Among the athletes was 44-year-old father and international shipbroker, Michael Wardian. In 2017, he set a record at the event by running all seven of the marathons under 2:55. This year, Wardian planned on tacking on three extra marathons at the end of the World Marathon Challenge in hopes of capturing the world record for the fastest completion of ten marathons in ten days.

Wardian is no stranger to these types of epic challenges. Just the month prior to his ten-marathon odyssey, he ran 27 straight hours to compete in the HURT 100 along the trails of the semi-tropical rainforest above Honolulu, one of the most grueling 100-mile courses on the planet. He also holds the record for the fastest Leadville Trail 100-mile race and Pikes Peak Marathon double and the fastest 50K on a treadmill. That's not to mention that he's qualified for and competed in three U.S. Olympic marathon trials.

Despite his pedigree, things almost immediately got off to a rocky start on the glacier in Novo. Having raced in Antarctica before, he expected temperatures to be colder. Instead, a 32-degree (0°C) day meant he started to sweat almost immediately. Even more troubling, though, was the fact that the terrain underfoot turned to mush. "It made it feel like running in sand," he would later tell me. Making matters worse, the wind picked up with fervor, whipping gusts of ice and snow in the faces of the runners. This left Wardian and his fellow runners to vacillate between overheating and fighting strong snow squalls, all while negotiating increasingly challenging footing. In his head, he debated whether he should waste time slowing down to

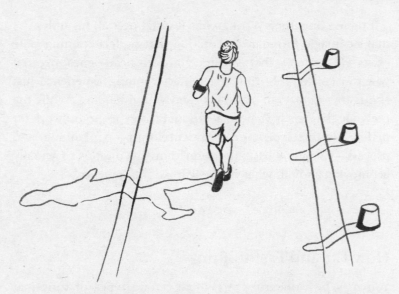

Approaching your runs with a mind of acceptance can help set the stage for flow.

shed a layer and when he should do it. Eventually, he told me, he commanded a stop to all the inner chatter:

> *"I just accepted the conditions and soon found myself moving with the course, rather than against it. I found lines I hadn't seen before, places to push the pace, and figured out how to navigate the headwinds and eventually I was moving. I wasn't pushing, but I was moving more and more ahead. I was just in the moment and that allowed me to release all expectations and flow."*

This was a turning point for him. Instead of fighting the elements, he employed a mind of acceptance, freeing up the headspace to enter that perfect running experience. He would end up crossing the finish line in first place wearing ski goggles and shorts in a time of 3:16:43.

If there's one thing Wardian has learned over all his miles, it's that no magic formula for entering that perfect running state exists. He contends that it's largely in your head—meaning that you can conceivably find the perfect running experience just about anywhere, even on an icy runway in Antarctica. While the previous chapters have been all about laying the groundwork for perfect running experiences—presence, purpose, planning, and process—Chapter 8 will offer some thoughts on how to actually get moving and put what you've learned into practice.

***

How Far and Fast to Run

You may be wondering: Are there certain types of runs that make perfect running experiences more likely? Do I have to run a specific pace, distance, or intensity? Where is the best place to run to facilitate optimal experiences? While there is still much we don't understand about optimal experiences, it's worth taking a look at the existing theories and research that give us clues.

Studies from the 1980s suggest that the runner's high generally develops around 25–35 minutes into a run. Thaddeus Kostrubala, M.D., a psychiatrist, researcher, and author once dubbed a "kind of high priest" of long-distance running, contended that after 30–40 minutes of running, an athlete could encounter a shift in consciousness. A more recent study involving ultramarathon runners measured brain activity via EEG every hour of a six-hour run, in addition to incrementally gauging cognitive performance, mood, and feelings of flow. After the first hour, they saw a significant boost in feelings of flow, but this decreased at subsequent check-ins over the next five hours. This suggests that a run likely has to be long enough that it gives time for your inner chatter to quiet down and for your body and brain to fall into sync. As you've seen in the stories in this book, however, optimal states of consciousness on the run can materialize at even the unlikeliest of times.

While most of the evidence suggests that some level of running intensity is required to induce flow, further research on the subject points to the fact that perfection is in the eye of the beholder and that it may take some trial and error for a runner to identify what types of runs cultivate greater feelings of perfection. One study published in *Medicine & Science in Sports & Exercise* that investigated the runner's high and gene expression theorized that the molecular switches within our RNA—which controls how genes are expressed in our cells—turn on in different ways, depending on the person and the type of run. So, while your running buddy can trigger the RNA pathways that lead to a runner's high with a hard and fast three-mile run, it might take you a two-hour steady state run.

Exercise 8.1: Perfect Post-Run Reflection

Reflecting on what conditions lead to perfect running experiences can help you get back to that headspace. Ask yourself the following questions:

- What factors set me up to experience a perfect run today?
- Were there outside forces that facilitated it?
- What did that perfect running state feel like?
- What adjustments should I make next time around?

In my experience, I regularly experience brushes with perfection on everyday runs of 4–5 miles with my dog—call it a runner's high, micro-flow, or fleeting transcendence. I don't need to be in the best shape of my life or even have any significant goal in mind. My most powerful perfect running experiences, however, have been in longer workouts or races when I'm pushing myself and have my sights set on a tangible objective, something more akin to what is described in the literature as the flow state.

In your search for perfect running, it's worth experimenting with the types of runs that invoke greater feelings of timelessness and joy. While every runner should work to incorporate a variety of workouts, it can be helpful to know which runs inspire greater levels of perfection.

* * *

Where to Run

Antarctica wasn't Michael Wardian's only encounter with perfection on his journey to complete the ten-marathon challenge. In fact, he reported entering that state multiple times in a variety of environments, even in the worst of circumstances. Upon leaving Novo, Wardian and the other runners flew back to Cape Town, where he handily won the second race in a time of 2:57:58. They flew on to run marathons in Perth, Australia, followed by Dubai, Madrid, and Santiago, Chile, all of which he won. In Santiago, he faced an unexpected hurdle that ultimately led him to an "ah ha" moment of sorts. He told me:

> *"I had stomach issues and I knew I didn't have enough energy to run my best, but I also knew that if I kept moving I would get it done. I was running around this tiny park in the middle of the night thinking, 'This is so cool, how many people will ever get to do this,' and that unlocked flow. I just started thinking how lucky I was to be there and I wanted to honor all the people who believed in me and sacrificed for me to get to do these things. Next thing I know, I am moving around super well and ended up kicking the sickness that was hampering me."*

In addition to his top finish in Santiago, he would go on to win the final race of the World Marathon Challenge in Miami, Florida, in a time of 2:53:03, making it a clean sweep. He followed that up with three more marathons near his home in Washington, D.C., setting the fastest average time for ten marathons in ten days: 2:55:17. What's more, he celebrated by tackling a 5K race on the eleventh day, running a 5:28-mile pace with his dog.

While Wardian's story demonstrates that flow can be found in all sorts of places, it's no coincidence that his strongest examples come from more natural locales. No matter what type of run you're doing, environmental factors play a major role in guiding your path toward that perfect running state. The takeaway is this: If you want to stack the odds in your favor, head out for a run in the great outdoors—the greener or bluer, the better. Whether it's a tree-lined city park, a forest trail, a windswept mountain, or an expanse of ocean real estate, there's something about being out in nature that inspires feelings of transcendence.

This is probably because we as human beings harbor a biological need to connect with nature. Indeed, for the vast majority of human existence, nature was our home. Pulitzer Prize-winning author and Harvard scientist Edward O. Wilson suggests that we are "hardwired" for that connection and that our health is inextricably linked to time spent in nature. He popularized the term "biophilia," which was originally coined by social psychologist Erich Fromm. The idea has inspired much research that reveals humans' innate draw to nature and the positive ways we respond to spending time in it.

Even the medical field has begun to awaken to this important connection. Doctors in Scotland's Shetland Islands issue "nature prescriptions" for chronic health issues and professionals in Japan tout the benefits of Shinrin-yoku or "forest bathing." This simply involves mindfully moving through a forested area while engaging the senses. At the Japanese Society of Forest Medicine, researchers examine the therapeutic effects on human health related to spending time in forests. They have discovered that it can reduce stress, anxiety, and depression, boost the immune system, and enhance cardiovascular and metabolic health. Other research found that forest bathing reduces cortisol levels, lowers heart rate and blood pressure, and calms the sympathetic nervous system.

Researchers in the UK sought to further make the distinction between the importance of not just being outside, but of spending time in more natural settings. To do this, they fitted a group of people with mobile electrodes on their heads and had them walk through three different environments: An urban shopping district, a park with ample green space, and a bustling commercial area. They discovered that when the participants walked through the park, their brain wave patterns shifted to a more relaxed state—reducing feelings of frustration and stress and promoting a more meditative mindset. Similarly, another study found that people's brain waves shifted to a more present-centered, meditative state when they went from a busy urban setting to a green space.

Exercise 8.2: Advice for City Slickers

The United Nations Population Division estimates that by 2050, three-quarters of the people on Earth will live in cities, so if your runs are mostly in an urban setting, you aren't alone. In urban areas you have to tune out distractions—cars honking, unpleasant smells, other pedestrians hurrying past. In nature, you are able to simply open up your senses and relax into the experience. With that said, most cities have wonderful trails and parks that not only provide uninterrupted stretches of real estate to run, they also ensure greater safety. Consider the following tricks for finding small slivers of nature in urban environments:

• Identify nearby parks and trail systems: Pull up a map on your phone and look for large green spaces or bodies of water. These geographic features are often accompanied by pedestrian walkways.

- Be strategic about choosing your routes: Work to locate routes that limit the number of stop lights and always make sure there are sidewalks in heavily trafficked areas to ensure greater safety.
- Run at less busy times of day: If you can make it work, avoid running during morning or afternoon rush hour when traffic is at its peak.
- Embrace the chaos: Finally, if you do most of your training in an urban jungle, work to find awe in the sights, sounds, and life of the cityscape. Inspiration can be discovered just about anywhere if you look for it.

Some of my most memorable perfect runs have been aided in large part by nature. One run in particular that stands out was in Joshua Tree National Park in southern California in 2018. Camping with a group of outdoor writers and editors, I snuck out of my single-person tent one morning as soon as the sun rose for a solo jaunt through the park. I pulled on my running shoes and headed down a dusty trail. As I ran, I was captivated by the way the light struck the imposing spike-leafed evergreens. Shards of the morning sun pierced through the trees on either side of the trail, flickering as I passed. Red cactus flowers dotted the horizon. Every few minutes I spotted a black-tailed jackrabbit running across my path or standing roadside with alert attention. The deserted landscape and windswept piles of bare rock and colossal boulders made it feel otherworldly.

Although I had no particular agenda for this run, I quickly fell into a rhythm, entranced by the immersive nature of the environment around me. Losing track of time, I ran further than intended before looping back to base camp. I felt almost giddy as my legs effortlessly carried me up the final climb to my tent. With no initial expectations, this next-level run took me by surprise.

Indeed, place not only changes the running experience, but running also changes the way you experience it. Your heart rate elevates, veins and capillaries dilate, there's an increase in the flow of oxygen to the muscles and brain, and endorphins enter the system. As a result, your perception of the landscape becomes more dynamic and you engage in a wholly unique form of kinetic empathy. When you run, spatial relationships are different than when you are inert or walking at a slower speed. The experience encompasses not just what you see visually, but the terrain you feel underfoot, the changes in air pressure, the direction of the wind, and the quality of the air.

What runners say

Many of the runners I surveyed identified off-road trails as being important to achieving that perfect running headspace, largely thanks to their focusing effect. Several mentioned that they struggled to find a rhythm when surrounded by too many outside distractions. Here's what some had to say.

"Sometimes road runs limit my ability to get in the zone, because I have to be focused on so many other factors— stop lights, uneven sidewalks, not getting hit by cars, etc."

Meg S, 29, Denver, CO

"I like to run in peaceful places—I am lucky to live close to the countryside. For me, environment plays a role in getting into the zone—that Zen state where mind and body just flow."

Amanda, H., 48, Droitwich, UK

"I think it helps when I'm on a single-track trail. My theory is that focusing on foot placement around rocks and roots is a way of keeping my mind focused on being in the moment. I also think it helps when I'm taking in the rest of my surroundings in a positive way, whether it's snow sparkling in the sun, warm rain dripping down my face, or beautiful wildflowers blooming—I could go on—I guess it's about being grateful and present with whatever environment you are running in."

Sarah H., 36, Jackson, WY

"Sometimes traffic both in the sense of cars, plus people and animals, makes it challenging to get in the zone. It's important to be aware of your surroundings, but I am often too observant and that can be a hard habit to break."

Phil B., 55, Basingstoke, Hampshire, UK

"Running downhill really helps, especially 'flowy' downhill paths like mountain bike trails."

Sylvia D., 28, El Portal, CA

"Frequent distractions interrupt flow—my dog pulling on the leash, encountering too many other people on an urban path, running too fast or too slow."

Ryan T., 26, Minneapolis, MN

"If you're dodging dogs and their walkers, kids on bikes, construction that blocks the sidewalk, then that can interrupt that flow-finding process."

John G., 40, Philadelphia, PA

As was mentioned in Chapter 3, a key component of the awe that is often experienced in nature is called "soft fascination." Soft fascination involves attention that requires little effort—maybe you notice the way the breeze is rustling the leaves on a tree or the ripple of the water as it flows down a gentle mountain stream. This keeps you engaged in the moment without requiring excess cognitive resources to maintain attention.

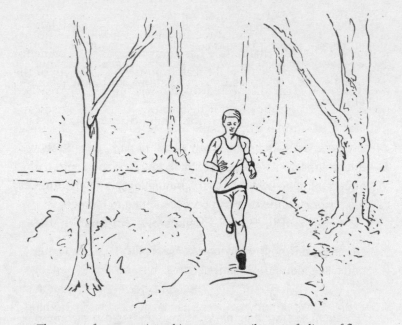

The sense of awe experienced in nature contributes to feelings of flow.

Research also shows that moving through nature leads to electrochemical changes in the brain that can help us enter a state of unforced attention. That sense of wonder that is experienced in nature can create deep moments of insight and realization of our place in the universe. If you've ever felt immersed in the moment at the peak of a mountain looking over a valley below or marveled at a spectacular expanse of ocean, you've experienced the seeds of optimal experience. When you're captured by nature, your focus narrows and you feel one with your surroundings. These are all flow-adjacent experiences and the ideal breeding ground for a perfect run.

It will come as no surprise that the experts have long argued that nature can be a contributor to flow. Optimal focus and attention are important aspects of any perfect run and the great outdoors has a way of improving both. In fact, "Attention Restoration

Theory" suggests that concentration is enhanced and we operate at our best when we spend time in the natural world. Another reason experts posit that nature has a way of setting the scene for flow is the fact that it offers a break from the busy reality of the everyday. One study discovered that flow is more easily reached when your surroundings limit distractions and offer an escape from the hustle and bustle of daily life. To be sure, natural settings are shown to be more intrinsically pleasurable to people, as well as more conducive to creating that sense of timelessness. All of these factors play in the favor of nature's role in making that perfect headspace more easily accessible.

Exercise 8.3: Finding Flow on the Treadmill

There's a good reason the treadmill has so many negative nicknames—The Dreadmill, The Hamster Wheel, Satan's conveyer belt—for many runners it can be deadly boring. Nothing throws a road block in front of a potentially perfect run like the monotony of running on a rotating belt in an austere gym or dark basement.

So, is finding flow possible on a treadmill? The answer is yes, although it's more challenging. My philosophy on treadmills is that they can be a great option for running when running outdoors isn't possible and a workout might otherwise be skipped. They assist in providing continuity in training and contributing to fitness that will ultimately boost your chances of achieving more perfect runs when you get back to outdoor running. Here are a few tips to help you find greater enjoyment on the treadmill. While it might not be anywhere near perfect, dread is not a requirement.

• Vary the incline: The tedium of treadmill running is partially due to the lack of terrain changes. Running on the same flat belt mile after mile can also contribute to repetitive stress injuries. So why not throw in a few hills? Increase the incline for longer or shorter hills periodically throughout your run to keep you engaged and work different muscles.

- Change up your speed: I often choose to throw in a number of surges on the treadmill, especially in the winter when I do less speed work outdoors. After a good warm-up, increase your speed for 30–60 seconds. Bring it back to an easier pace for several minutes and then do another surge. Repeat several times and be sure to cool down at the end.
- Work on form: The treadmill offers a unique opportunity to scrutinize your form. Not only can you keep pace and terrain constant, you will have fewer environmental distractions. Pick a pace that is difficult enough that you could utter a few words here and there, but can't easily hold an entire conversation. Pay attention to the way you carry your arms, your posture, how your knees drive forward, and how your feet hit the belt. Consider having a friend take a video of you from the side, front, and back to get a better idea of what your stride looks like.
- Always bring a water bottle: Since indoor air is often dry and you'll sweat more without a breeze, take advantage of the perk of a designated water bottle holder on the treadmill.

In the end, even when you purposefully select training environments and workouts that are meant to induce running perfection, it doesn't always arise. To be sure, part of the thrill of entering this transcendent state is its mystery. As a coach, I tell athletes to focus on "controlling the controllables." This simply means that while there is value in working to regulate things within your wherewithal, devoting energy to worrying about factors outside of your control is less productive.

Wardian says that even for a professional ultrarunner like himself, running isn't all flowy euphoria. During his ten-marathon journey, he contends that some days felt like a fruitless grind. It was enduring those moments, though, that eventually made way for next-level breakthroughs. He explained:

"I was able to find periods during many of the ten marathons where I reached a flow state, but there were also a lot of the races where it was a grunt and I just had to put my head down and do the work. That is what I love about running, there are no shortcuts or guarantees. You either do or you don't and, sure, there are circumstances that can affect those outcomes, but running is very true and I appreciate and respect that."

Now that we've covered some theories on how to put the principles of perfect running into motion, Chapter 9 will look at those times when you feel stuck and unable to cultivate perfect running, as well as offering thoughts on the importance of letting go and allowing those perfect runs to come to you, rather than becoming obsessed with chasing them down.

Practices in Perfection

- Perfect runs arise amid all types of runs.
- For that flowy state to arise, the run has to be long enough to allow the mental chatter to quiet, but not so long that you're distracted by fatigue and discomfort.
- Different types of runs can lead to different levels of the perfect running experience.
- Running in nature changes the way you view the experience of a run, but running itself also alters the way you view nature.

CHAPTER 9
FINDING PERFECTION IN IMPERFECTION

"Flow can't be forced, because force is met with a counter force. Flow is something that has to happen without tension or pushing."

THE MORNING OF the women's marathon at the 2004 Olympics in Athens, headlines were dominated by a single theme: Heat. Temperatures hung in the triple digits and high humidity made the air feel downright sweltering—far from ideal for a grueling 26.2-mile race from the historic town of Marathon to Athens.

On account of the conditions, American Deena Kastor planned for a slow start. Committed to keeping a conservative pace and running her own race, she watched the leaders— superstars Paula Radcliffe of Britain and Catherine Ndereba of Kenya among them—pull away in the early miles. She reminded herself to hold back and focus on taking in fluids, cooling herself with saturated sponges, and running in the patches of shade whenever possible.

By the halfway point, though, the leaders pulled away out of sight, a full two minutes ahead of Kastor. She mindfully did a head-to-toe inventory, checking for signs of overheating and dehydration. She picked up the pace ever so slightly, working to reel back in her competitors. As far back as 18th place at one point, she began picking runners off one by one. First Italy. Then China. Then Russia.

She ran with smooth precision, adeptly scaling more than 700 feet (213 meters) of altitude from miles 11 through 19 (17.7–30.5 km). Falling into a rhythm, she listened to her feet hitting the warm, freshly laid tarmac as the sun set and the punishing heat of the day dissipated. Lights on either side of the road flickered on as she passed the Panathenaic Stadium and the Olympic flame. She overtook Japanese, Ethiopian, and Serbian runners. Feeling light and fast, she moved quickly past Ethiopia's Elfenesh Alemu with less than a mile to go.

"I was definitely in a flow state of running the second half of the Athens Olympic Marathon," she recalled to me in 2019. "I remember picking up the pace and passing people, yet I wasn't feeling restricted with the great effort. My last mile clocked at 4:45 and I felt as if I could have run that fast forever."

When she entered the Panathenaic Stadium, the site of the first modern Olympics in 1896, her stride lengthened and her arms pumped. Crossing the finish line in 2:27:20, she captured the bronze medal and became the first American woman to medal in the event since its inception in 1984.

While Kastor has experienced her fair share of flow-driven, mountaintop moments like the one in Athens, she insists that they are the exception. "Trying to improve at anything takes a long stretch outside your comfort level," she told me. "I would estimate that my own training and racing is about 95 percent effort—either mental or physical—and 5 percent flow or bliss. The struggle is so worth it."

To be sure, Kastor's story underscores the rule of perfection, which is that it is found in imperfection and struggle. She says that those perfect days, like the one at the 2004 Olympics, only come through practice and persistence. "Then your body adapts and maybe the stars align and you have an effortful, yet effortless day of running," she said. This final chapter is all about how to stick with running through the struggle to eventually put you on

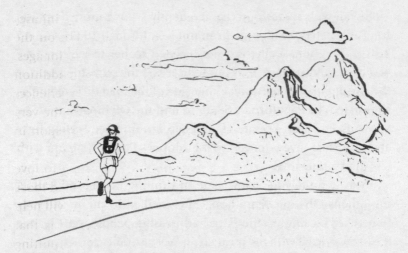

Every run won't be perfect, but persistence over time offers great pay offs.

a path toward perfection. As Kastor insists, playing the long game and accepting the highs and lows of the running life is what will get you there.

***

What to Do When Perfection Feels Out of Reach

Sometimes there is no "high," no feeling of being one with the universe, no sensation you are effortlessly running at breakneck pace. Sometimes your feet hurt and your back aches and you feel like you're going to throw up. Sometimes one mile feels like ten and frustration and defeat set in.

Every runner experiences bad runs and dips in motivation—those times when you just feel stuck. Maybe you woke up one day and suddenly felt like running was the last thing you wanted to do. Or perhaps you've been struggling with incessant injuries and every time you restart training, you end up back on the bench. Or maybe you've been trying to get into running for ages, but can't find the inspiration to stick with training. In addition to turning running into a joyless grind, these experiences eliminate the possibility of encountering perfect runs, the very thing that has the potential to inspire a real love of the sport in the first place.

If this sounds like you, first remember: It's okay not to love every step of training. In fact, it's important to understand that's completely normal. While it is my hope that this book will help you discover more joyful days of running, the reality is that some runs will still be about simply showing up and putting in the mileage. Continuing to push isn't always the right thing to do, but successful training requires a level of commitment to running that involves logging miles when you don't always feel like it.

I often liken it to writing—I don't wake up wholly excited to put words on the page every single day, but the purposeful practice of doing so allows for breakthroughs and flow experiences down the road. In fact, it is often just on the other side of struggle that perfection begins to miraculously materialize. As I discussed in the introduction to this book, the type of perfection we're talking about here is not of flawlessness—the origins of perfection lie in the unification of seemingly imperfect factors. Struggle is a necessary part of any long and satisfying career. It's what makes the transcendent moments—those perfect runs—that much more meaningful when you do encounter them.

Of course, there are also instances when you feel stuck and the best course of action is to hang up your running shoes for a few days or weeks and (gasp!) quit. Those include things like overtraining, injuries, illness, mental burnout, and post-race recovery and will be addressed in the following pages. A simple loss of motivation, though, doesn't necessarily signal that you need to back off of training. Keep in mind that the lack of inspiration to run that I'm referring to is different than a general lack of motivation to get out of bed and do other things you normally enjoy. This might signal a more serious condition. In those cases, be sure to consult a medical expert to help get you back on track. This chapter is simply meant to provide "quick hits" on how to identify problems and get you up and running during periods of waning inspiration—to set you up to eventually experience more perfect runs. If you've lost your running mojo, consider some of the following reasons runners get stuck, as well as potential solutions.

Reason #1: Training isn't going as planned
When you struggle to reach performance or fitness goals, it can feel like you're banging your head against the wall. Even when you think you're doing everything right, runners often encounter frustrating plateaus in performance or stagnation in fitness.

Try this: Remember that progress takes time. As they say, patience is a virtue. These plateaus can usually be overcome with simple changes to training. If your body has adapted to your current regimen, you may need to change things up and add new workouts into your weekly running calendar.

Reason #2: You keep getting injured
There's nothing like one ailment after the next to kill motivation to train. If your injury status has become a game of whack-a-mole, it's time to reassess your approach to training. Indeed, one minor issue that goes unaddressed can cascade into a long list of other related problems.

Try this: In addition to connecting with a coach to talk training, you may also want to consult a medical professional. No matter how much you tweak training or back off of running, these injuries are likely to return if you don't address the root cause. A doctor or physical therapist can prescribe changes in training, supplemental exercises, and cross-training activities.

Reason #3: You've lost sight of your goals and purpose

Maybe your reasons to run—your goals, intentions, and mission statement—were all clear at the outset of training, but over months and years of running, you've lost sight of them. A general lack of direction in training can leave a runner feeling aimless and without motivation to get out the door. It can also mean that day-to-day training is somewhat haphazard, making it hard for you to buy into your program and understand why you're doing what you're doing.

Try this: The go-to solution for this problem is to sign up for a race. A big event on the horizon has a way of injecting a new sense of enthusiasm into training. On a more existential level, if you have set goals, but continue to feel adrift in your training, you should go back to your running mission statement and work on refining it. Runners will frequently find that the purpose behind their running changes depending on the season of training and life they are in. Spend time reflecting on your reason to run and how your daily training aligns with that purpose.

Reason #4: You're bored

Boredom is an oft-cited complaint among people just starting to run, but it can also strike the most experienced of harriers. The majority of your runs should feel like fresh and new experiences, so if training has become more of a slog, you know the tedium of an uninspired running routine has taken hold.

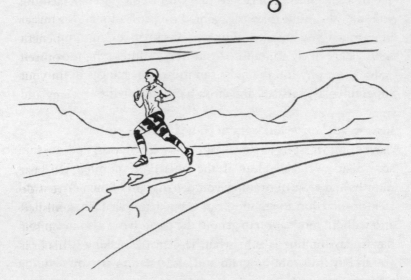

Identifying the things that contribute to and detract from your motivation to run is essential.

Try this: Many runners make the mistake of running the same route, distance, and pace day after day. If lethargy has set in, it's time to mix things up. This might mean scouring the internet for new workout ideas, identifying a new training environment, joining a running club, or swapping a day of running for a cross-training activity.

Reason #5: You're distracted

Motivation is hindered when running feels burdensome, like another thing you have to cram into an already busy day. While it may have started as a pursuit of recreation, competition, or self-care, the joy of running can quickly get lost when it begins to feel like a chore and you're constantly training in a state of distraction.

Try this: Work on reframing running in your mind—as something you get to do, rather than are required to do. To be sure, the busier you are in other areas of life, the more likely it is you'll benefit from setting aside a little time each day to run. Remind yourself that rather than taking time away from other priorities in your life, running can enhance them by giving you greater energy and emotional equilibrium.

Reason #6: You've become too competitive
Whether you're gunning for a personal best or racing to beat your arch-rival, becoming consumed by the competitive side of the sport can eventually lead to frustration and diminished motivation. You know you've got an issue if you find yourself obsessed by certain goals both on and off the running trails or if you're overly upset by lackluster workouts or races.

Try this: Reflect on what's driving your competitive nature. Is it jealousy, a deep need to prove yourself to others, a feeling of inadequacy, a tendency to constantly compare yourself? When you get to the root of your competitive motivations, you might find they signal a larger issue. If this is the case, ask yourself if your obsession with achievements is productive and if you might be able to redirect that energy toward more sustainable intentions and pursuits.

Reason #7: You're under pressure to perform
Feeling undue pressure to perform can quickly take the joy out of training. This involves being preoccupied with pleasing outside parties like a coach or family member. Outside pressure tends to make it difficult to remain present in the day-to-day practice of running, which often has a detrimental effect on performance.

Try this: Work on harnessing the mindfulness skills discussed in Chapter 3. When you're feeling under pressure, reflect on your own personal reasons to run. While you might not be able to defuse the source of the stress, your mindset and direction of focus is within your control.

Reason #8: Time of Year
There's a reason you will see hordes of runners joyfully bounding down the running trails on a sunny 60-degree day and hardly anyone out there when the snow falls and the temperatures drop. Weather can be a major source of inspiration or the lack thereof.

Try this: Come up with a plan for how you will adjust training with the seasons of the year. For instance, if you live in an area with a snowy winter, your focus may be simply to maintain fitness. Weather can also offer a natural excuse to work in some additional cross-training during certain months of the year, so come spring, your legs and mind feel fresh and ready to run.

* * *

Reasons You May Need Time Away from Training

Never quit. Never give up. These are some of the most common sentiments uttered in the sports arena. Sometimes though, quitting is exactly what you should do. Part of being a successful athlete is having the intuition to know when to throw in the towel. If you've tried some of the aforementioned solutions to no avail, it may be time to step away from running for a number of days, weeks, or even months.

"If you find your workouts are getting stagnant and your excitement for running is dwindling, it's not that you're necessarily doing anything wrong, you probably just need a break," coach

Tony Ruiz told me. "When an athlete starts to get concerned that they haven't been feeling good and they've been encountering little injuries one after the other, I immediately think they might need a 7–10 day break from running. Ninety-five percent of the time, a well-timed break will keep you from encountering a major injury or burnout."

While there are plenty of good reasons to back off of training, the five non-negotiable scenarios are as follows: Overtraining, injury, illness, mental burnout, and post-race. After taking some time off, you'll reenter training fresh and primed for more of those perfect runs. As with everything in this book, I always suggest you visit your doctor for approval on individual training practices and decisions.

Overtraining

Overtraining syndrome involves multiple body systems, including the nervous system, the endocrine system (hormones), and the immune system. Symptoms often include fatigue, unexplained illness, elevated heart rate, muscle soreness, insomnia, and negative changes in mood and motivation, along with reduced performance. The cause of overtraining is straightforward: Not enough rest in the context of training. With that said, the symptoms of anemia can be similar, so it may be worth ruling that out by having your doctor do a simple blood test.

All types of runners experience overtraining. Whether you're a new runner who is increasing mileage too quickly or an elite athlete trying to complete too many high-intensity workouts without enough recovery days, constantly overreaching in the fitness department can spell trouble. Overreaching involves increasing training load and inducing a state of temporary fatigue. Done strategically, it can take you to new levels of performance, but continual overreach is a recipe for burnout.

Many runners are overachievers who have trouble letting go of the idea that if some training is good, more is better. If you experience the symptoms associated with overtraining, it's time to rest. For some athletes, completely backing off training might be necessary. For others, it may mean logging light mileage for a couple of weeks. In either case, it's likely you'll sacrifice some fitness, but it's the only way to reestablish your body's equilibrium.

Injury

Running injuries come in many shapes and sizes. Some are acute, while others are due to overuse, the latter being the most common in runners. Acute ailments occur when you, say, sprain your ankle on rough terrain or pull a muscle during a fast sprint. Overuse injuries, however, are the cumulative effect of repeated stress. These usually start small, but when they go unaddressed, become much worse.

Research suggests that upward of 70 percent of runners sustain an overuse injury during any given year. Some of the most common examples of these types of ailments in the running population are stress fractures, shin splints, plantar fasciitis, patellar tendonitis, IT band syndrome, and Achilles tendonitis. As with overtraining, the rehabilitation protocol will depend on the individual runner. In many cases, injuries necessitate time off of running. Often, athletes are cleared to continue to engage in low-impact cross-training activities that don't exacerbate the injury, but allow them to maintain some level of fitness.

Illness

Not all illnesses require time away from training, so it's important to employ good body awareness to know when you should back off. Many runners will train through minor head colds, but depending on how you're feeling, you may want to at least reduce your mileage and intensity. More serious issues, like upper respiratory illnesses, fever, various infections, the flu, and gastrointestinal issues call for rest. In these instances, it is important to allow your body to allocate resources toward fighting off the illness and recovering. Not only does research show that hard running can temporarily compromise the immune system, taking time off to let your body heal will actually get you back to regular training sooner than trying to run through illness.

Mental burnout

Mental burnout is sometimes a symptom of overtraining, but it can also strike all on its own. It's generally characterized by a feeling of being stale and "checked out" of training. I like to call it "the blahs." A runner who is experiencing psychological burnout may have trouble focusing during a workout or can barely even muster up the energy to start a run in the first place. Once you've ruled out physical issues causing this (a deficiency, for instance), you can look at the psychological side of the equation. Research shows that mental fatigue negatively impacts physical performance, proving it's not something you can just muscle through. Mental burnout makes running feel harder, even if you haven't increased distance, speed or intensity. For runners experiencing this, not only is rest important, but also engaging in other non-running-related activities. Try stepping back from worrying about your fitness and give your brain a break from the constant push of training.

Post-race

Most coaches prescribe anywhere from one to three weeks off of running after a big goal race to allow the body to heal. Sometimes this can involve light training, but for the most part, taking a

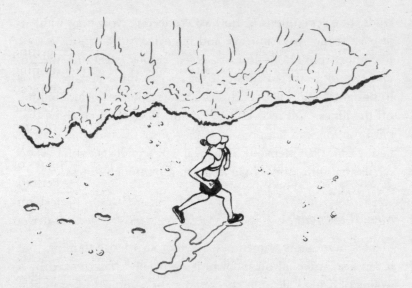

Rest and recovery are essential, no matter your pace, experience, or ambitions.

couple of weeks away from running is good for both body and mind. This is often difficult for runners following a race when adrenaline and enthusiasm are high, but consider this: Research shows that in the seven days following a marathon, skeletal muscle cells remain in necrosis, which involves the death of living cells and tissue. Even if you raced a shorter distance, the body needs time to recover.

This doesn't mean that you can't engage in other types of exercise. In fact, once your body has had a few days to bounce back, it's a great time to try something new or enjoy activities that were put on the back burner during training. As you begin running again, be sure to approach training conservatively. A couple of weeks of easy running is usually a good way to ease back in before kicking off another training cycle.

***

Learning to Let Go

Harboring a mindset of acceptance is essential to getting unstuck and cultivating the right conditions for perfect running experiences to arise, whether this means letting go of pushing so hard in training to allow an injury to heal, letting go of unrealistic goals to focus on new ones, letting go of a bad performance to refocus on the next race, letting go of preconceived plans to find peace in taking unscheduled time off, or just letting go of expectations to allow yourself to run for the joy of it. Perhaps most importantly, letting go of the pursuit of the perfect run must occur if you hope to discover healthy and flow-driven running.

Consider the sentiments Deena Kastor offered me: "Flow can't be forced, because force is met with a counter force. Flow is something that has to happen without tension or pushing." Neuroscientist Leslie Sherlin said something similar: "You can absolutely set yourself up to experience flow. If I'm being truly mindful, I'm not aspiring to experience flow, I am simply accepting where I'm at. If I'm chasing flow, I'm unlikely to experience it."

Even when we understand this on an intellectual level, however, human beings can be control freaks. Runners often think that if they follow training to the letter, eat right, get enough sleep, and buy the right shoes, goals are all but ensured to be fulfilled. In the same way, some become preoccupied with the idea of experiencing the perfect run, believing that a special formula will elicit the state at will.

To be sure, our tendency is to choose action over inaction, something behavioral scientists call "commission bias." We always feel we need to do something—anything—to thrust progress forward. This leads us to push for results through sheer force of will when the situation calls for patience and perseverance. What is the result of these natural human tendencies? Attachment. We become attached to all sorts of outcomes—setting a personal best in a race, running a flawless workout, logging a certain number of miles, outrunning a rival, or losing a certain number of pounds. You can even become attached to the idea of the perfect running experience.

When you become overly attached to an outcome, you have basically decided that without achieving it, you won't be happy. This tight grip on certain goals can cause a runner to take foolish actions—to run through an injury or continue training when on the verge of sickness. On the level of professional athletics, attachment is what leads athletes to dope and take other unethical actions in attempts to control outcomes.

So how do we overcome the human tendency to control and cling to our goals? First, it's important to distinguish the difference between attachment, detachment, and non-attachment. Take this example: You're training for a marathon in hopes of running a Boston qualifying time. The Boston Marathon is known to be one of the most challenging races to gain entry into. A "BQ" is determined by age and gender—and even if you run a qualifying time, there's a cap on the number of participants. As a result, thousands of runners who technically qualify don't get in each year.

To better your chances, you hire a coach and set forth an ambitious training plan. All is going according to plan three months into training. You're logging the best workouts and highest miles of your life. Then one day, you feel a minor pain in your knee during a workout. Instead of slowing down to examine it, you push through because you know it is a key training session.

That evening you find yourself experiencing greater discomfort and limping slightly. Despite worsening pain and a hitch in your gait, the next day you run again and the day after that you log another hard workout. You're terrified at the thought of skipping any training and taking time off to heal because that might mean you have to abandon or adjust your goal. You're stressed, tense, and in pain. This scenario is the result of an unhealthy attachment to a specific outcome—running a Boston qualifier. Attachment has inspired a death grip on the original training plan, clouding your judgment, preventing adjustments, and causing further injury.

On the other hand, consider an alternative response: When you feel that pain in your knee, you stop running immediately and head home. Rather than consulting your coach or pursuing medical advice, you simply hang up your running shoes for a few weeks and go about your business. You tell yourself you aren't disappointed, nor do you care all that much about how this may affect your marathon performance. This is detachment.

Psychologists often refer to this behavior as "emotional avoidance" (EA). It's characterized by an emotional defensiveness that keeps you from becoming too invested in an outcome in an attempt to subvert uncomfortable thoughts and emotions. In the end, this type of detachment is a form of escapism and eventually leads to psychological suffering when those repressed emotions inevitably rise to the surface of your psyche.

Neither attachment nor detachment is a healthy approach when it comes to training and goal attainment. The path that leads to more perfect running is underscored by an attitude of acceptance of the process of training and racing. Acceptance involves putting forth hopes, dreams, and goals, but also recognizing that everything isn't in your control. You care about the outcome and will do your best to achieve it, but some things you simply have to let go. Acceptance is characterized by non-attachment. This frame of mind inspires a recognition that growth can result even when things don't go according to plan— remember, perfection is found through the coming together of seemingly imperfect factors—making it a prerequisite for genuine experience.

The Buddhist parable of the "second arrow" offers an apt illustration of what acceptance is all about. In the previous example the first arrow is the oncoming knee injury. That pain in your knee hurts in the physical sense, but also on a deeper psychological level. It likely means that you will need to take some time off of training, potentially putting your goal of running a Boston qualifier at risk. Someone who is overly attached to their goal may fight the reality they are faced with: They are going to keep running despite just being hit with the arrow of injury. That's when they incur the second arrow, which is the destructive reaction to the first arrow. In this case, that second arrow is stress, anxiety, and worsening injury.

Conversely, the detached runner tries to ignore the first arrow and pretend that they don't notice it or care about how it might affect their race plans. That runner also gets hit with a second arrow, which is characterized by the suffering that results from repressing emotions and separating oneself from reality.

With the practice of non-attachment, you accept the blow of the first arrow and then figure out what the next best move is. In this case, it is likely to go see a doctor and figure out rehabilitation and cross-training strategies that might help you address the injury and adjust training. Instead of catastrophizing what that pain in your knee might mean and clinging to your goal or pretending that you don't care about the result, you accept reality and move on. This allows you to dodge the pain of that second arrow and increases your chances of getting training back on track.

From an objective standpoint, the concepts of acceptance, non-attachment, and letting go makes sense, but how do you practice it when you are in the crosshairs of an arrow in order to make way for more perfect running experiences? Michael Wardian offered me these thoughts:

> *"Of all the ways I have found to enter the flow state, the one that works the most consistently for me is allowing my body and mind to find their rhythm and to not force it. It is like trying to make yourself fall asleep, the harder you want to sleep the harder it is to sleep, but if you just release the tension and get out the way, your body and mind find what they are looking for. I know it sounds easy, but sharpening that ability to move aside is tough, especially if you have big goals and want to accomplish incredible things, but if you have done the work and your mind is ready, I think sometimes standing aside and letting things happen can be the best way to get to where you want to go."*

While there are many roads to achieving a mind of non-attachment, two of the most important tools that will bolster your ability to wield acceptance are psychological flexibility and self-compassion. Similar to running fitness, these are skills that take time and practice to nurture.

Psychological Flexibility

Psychological flexibility is a measure of how readily a person adapts to changing situational demands, how effectively they shift perspective, and how well they balance the various wants and needs of life. The science of neuroplasticity shows that we can train our brains to respond to certain stimuli in specific ways that increase psychological flexibility and decrease suffering.

For good reason, this is a skill that is often discussed in the context of mindfulness-based approaches in the field of mental health, like Acceptance and Commitment Therapy and Mindfulness-

Based Cognitive Therapy. It is also something most coaches identify as key to good running performance. "Psychological flexibility plays a huge role in a runner's success, particularly over the long term," coach Ben Rosario told me. "During the course of a runner's career there will inevitably be ups and downs. Handling the downs, especially, can be quite challenging. You have to be able to roll with the punches."

A psychologically flexible person is one who operates consciously in the present moment and responds to things according to a rooted set of values and beliefs despite conflicting emotions and circumstances. In the case of the runner looking to punch their ticket to the Boston Marathon, psychological flexibility would lead them to examine the reality of the oncoming injury, understand that promptly addressing unexpected injuries contributes to a long and successful running career, and respond appropriately. Conjuring more perfect running experiences requires a similar mindset. While there are certain things you can do to cultivate the right conditions, many of which are mentioned in this book, at some point you need to simply step back and let training unfold with a mentality of acceptance.

Psychological flexibility can help you establish a mindset that emphasizes the long game, allowing for an acceptance of setbacks and challenges and a greater focus on process. Indeed, Rosario added, "The way I nurture that ability in the runners I work with is to get out in front of it and remind them that those challenging times will be a part of the process at some point. And then it's a matter of dealing with them in a practical manner."

The opposite—psychological inflexibility—leads to attachment behavior and avoidance strategies that can lead a person to get caught up in more suffering. Research shows that poor psychological flexibility is associated with anxiety, depression, reduced performance, and diminished well-being. Indeed, flexibility allows us to appreciate the powers of acceptance and be more deliberate in our response to life's stressors and unpredictabilities. In effect, it's a skill that literally makes it possible to "go with the flow."

Exercise 9.1: How to Improve Psychological Flexibility

How adaptive are you? Can you bend and flex when an arrow comes your way? This is a practice that takes training before it becomes second nature.

One of the drivers behind psychological inflexibility is a desire for control. Anything unknown that goes off script can make a person uncomfortable because it may alter the outcome. To manage this, becoming adept at recognizing other outcomes that can contribute to success is essential. This means subverting catastrophic thinking—the tendency to assume the worst possible outcome. In recognizing other potential outcomes, one begins to see that the worst-case scenario is often quite unlikely.

For our aforementioned aspiring Boston Marathon qualifier, instead of immediately assuming that any break in training will spell disaster for their goals, they might write down other possible scenarios that will occur from this unexpected knee pain. Here are some examples of how this might play out.

- I will cut this workout short and go home and ice my knee. If it still hurts tomorrow, I'll take a day or two off. Hopefully after a couple days away from training, the pain will have disappeared and I can pick up where I left off.
- I will cut this workout short and go to the doctor. They might discover I have tendonitis and suggest I take a couple weeks off of running, but tell me I can cross-train. I could ride the

stationary bike and swim for those two weeks and return to training without any major loss in fitness.

- I will cut this workout short and go to the doctor. They might discover I have a stress fracture and need to take several months off of training. I could go home and look at my calendar for next year and find that while I might have to put off my goal for another season, it will allow me a longer buildup in training to hopefully avoid any injuries next time around.

Even in the third "worst–case" scenario, which is arguably the most unlikely, psychological flexibility allows a runner to view the glass as half full. Quite often, runners discover that in hindsight, these injuries and unexpected layoffs, if responded to appropriately, lead to better results down the line.

Self-Compassion

While self-compassion was discussed in Chapter 4 as an important skill in forming your running narrative, it's also a key player in building a mind of acceptance. Self-compassion is distinct from self-esteem, which is largely concerned with how we evaluate ourselves in various situations and areas of life. Notably, self-compassion does not hinge on evaluation or judgment. Studies have shown that while self-compassion is inversely correlated with self-comparison and social physique anxiety, it is positively linked to intrinsic motivation. What's more, it has been shown to help combat the fear of failure in sport. Catastrophic thinking is a close cousin of fear of failure, so by avoiding this mindset, one is set up to productively accept the myriad of outcomes that can result in any given training cycle.

It is important to note that self-compassion isn't about giving yourself infinite slack. It is not generally associated with, for instance, letting yourself off the hook for repeatedly skipping

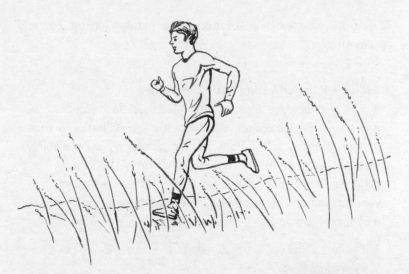

Harbouring self-compassion can help you better accept the inherent ups and downs of the running life.

runs to go to happy hour after work. It is different than self-indulgence, which puts you at the whims of your desire for immediate gratification. In fact, research has shown that self-compassion may actually enhance a person's motivation for self-improvement.

Self-criticism is the other side of this coin. Runners who tend toward perfectionism harbor little self-compassion in the face of setbacks. Rosario described this to me when he said the following: "Runners are often their own worst critics. Usually their criticism comes as a result of not hitting a certain time goal. I think that is a dangerous way to critique oneself. I would rather see runners assess themselves based on their effort, both in the short term after a race and in the long term." To be sure, lofty goals can be set with the understanding that unexpected forces outside of your control can knock you off course. Rather than criticizing oneself, research suggests that being compassionate is a more effective way of accepting reality, letting go, and reorienting.

Exercise 9.2: Cultivating Self-Compassion

A critical inner voice fires up feelings associated with distress and threat via increased activity in the sympathetic nervous system, whereas self-compassion can bolster a person's ability to remain calm in stressful situations by turning off that fight-or-flight response. Think of the ways that you use self-criticism in your training and racing. Begin by writing those down. Here are a couple of examples:

• If I didn't wimp out the final mile of the race, I would have run a personal best.
• I am often too lazy to run with the fast group in track workouts.

Then work to flip the script by jotting down a kinder way of framing each scenario.

• If I run a more even pace throughout my race, I'll have a better chance at running a personal best.
• If I try starting with the fast group in track workouts, maybe I will find I'm faster than I think.

This exercise can help you identify the ways your inner "tough love" is bringing you down and how a simple change in language can lead to a more motivated mindset.

Greater psychological flexibility and self-compassion in training can go a long way toward helping you accept the ups and downs of the running life. By approaching each episode of your training with a mind of acceptance, even in the moments you feel most stuck, you set yourself up for discovering more of those perfect running experiences down the road.

Practices in Perfection

- Some of the top reasons runners lose their running mojo are as follows: Training isn't going as planned, you encounter a string of injuries, you've lost sight of your goals and purpose, you're bored, you're distracted, you've become too competitive, you're under pressure to perform, and unfavorable weather.
- Every runner encounters times when they feel less motivated to run. In the case of overtraining, injury, illness, mental burnout, or after a race, you should back off of running for a number of days, weeks, or months.
- Always consult a medical professional at the outset of training, as well as when you run into physical or mental ailments.
- Learning to let go of pushing toward a specific end goal is key to facilitating perfect running experiences.
- Psychological flexibility and self-compassion can help you let go and find acceptance.

EPILOGUE

THROUGHOUT THIS BOOK we've seen perfect runs occur in all manner of situations and circumstances: At the top of a mountain in the Pyrenees after days of running, on a country road in Northern Minnesota on an easy run, on an icy airfield in Antarctica during a ten-marathon challenge, along a hurricane-soaked stretch of highway in North Carolina amid a 1,000-mile journey, on a muddy forest trail in Sweden during a four-year-long stint living in the woods, and en route to winning the Boston Marathon.

Running rarely serves up perfection on a silver platter. Staying the course over time on a less than perfect path is essential. Indeed, perfect running shouldn't be complicated. In terms of guiding principles for training, the top expert in the physiology of human endurance we met in Chapter 3, Dr. Michael Joyner, offers this clever haiku:

Run a lot of miles
Some faster than your race pace
Rest once in a while

We've discussed the ways approaching running as an activity that employs both a spirit of work and play can set the stage for optimal experiences on the run. In addition, we've examined the four main factors that contribute to perfect running: Presence, purpose, planning, and process. Above all, though, after researching, reporting, and writing this book, the only true conclusion I've come to is that letting the perfect run come to you is your surest path toward it. It's all about setting the stage and allowing the mystery of transcendence to unfold in its own time.

This may be somewhat unsatisfying for a running populace who tends to be interested in action, but consider this: While you can't will the perfect run into existence, when it does materialize, it forges new pathways in the brain that make it easier to find your way back to that special state of mind. What's more, these experiences have a way of not only imbuing your running with greater joy and meaning, but also having an influence well beyond the trails and tracks.

It is through the amalgamation of imperfect episodes of running that perfection arises. Of course, life is no different. Perfection can be found all around. All that it requires is for you to notice when the celestial bodies align to create something special—it's as simple and as complicated as remaining present and listening to your in-and-out breath and the left-right-left of your feet as you glide over the trail.

ACKNOWLEDGMENTS

My deepest gratitude to all the runners, coaches, and scientists who shared their stories with me. While I've been a runner nearly my entire life, you've extended my understanding of this sport that proves to be powerful for so many.

To my editors at Bloomsbury, especially Matthew Lowing. Always keen on smart collaboration, it was through our meeting of the minds that my ideas about *The Perfect Run* solidified. This book is better thanks to your guidance.

Gratitude is owed to the publications to which I contribute. Some of the insights and stories I recount in this book originated in columns for these publications. I feel fortunate every day to get to do the work I do.

Many thanks go to my willing first readers, especially my dad, Ted Lobby. You put me in my first pair of running shoes decades ago and have remained my greatest supporter every step of the way. And to my wonderful in-laws, John and Ann. Your support means the world to me.

To my family and our messy house, muddy footprints, middle-of-the-night snuggle sessions, and ice-cream dinners. Amid the joyful chaos that characterizes this season of life, you remind me every day of the perfection that is our beautiful mess. Welly, my loyal canine companion, you remain by my side, snout on keyboard, during the long and arduous days of book writing and pregnancy, never hesitating to pull me out the door for a run no matter how slow the miles get. Liesl, my firstborn, you are the brightest of lights in my life. Thank you for reminding me what's really important—I'll always be ready to take my feet outside with you. Liv, you bumped around in my belly throughout the entire writing of this book. I can think of no greater inspiration.

And to Jason, my partner on this adventure, an equal co-parent and leader of our girl squad, an editor and sounding board during exhaustive months of writing, my favorite running partner, and a shoulder to cry on and love to laugh with. I love you guys to the moon and back. You are all perfect to me.

ABOUT THE AUTHOR

Mackenzie L. Havey is the author of *Mindful Running* (Bloomsbury, 2017). She writes about endurance sports, mind/body health and wellness, and adventure travel for *Runner's World, SELF, Triathlete, TheAtlantic.com, ESPN.com, OutsideOnline.com* and elsewhere. In addition to completing 14 marathons and an Ironman triathlon, she is a USA Track & Field-certified coach, an instructor in the Physical Activity Program in the School of Kinesiology at the University of Minnesota and has done training in Mindfulness-Based Stress Reduction. She studied English at the College of St. Benedict and has a master's in kinesiology with an emphasis in sport and exercise psychology from the University of Minnesota. She lives with her husband, two young daughters, and vizsla in Minneapolis.

MLHavey.com

RESOURCES

Introduction

pursuit of perfection has risen ... Curran, T. and Hill, A. P. (2019). "Perfectionism is increasing over time: A meta-analysis of birth cohort differences from 1989 to 2016." *Psychological Bulletin*, 145(4), 410–429.

dates back to antiquity ... According to the ancient philosopher and poet Empedocles (*c*. 495–435 BCE), perfection could only be found in imperfection.

It's a feeling ... McMillan, G. Author interview 4 February 2019.

centerpiece of a satisfying life ... Peterson, C., Park, N. and Seligman, M.E.P. (2005). "Orientations to happiness and life satisfaction: The full life versus the empty life." *Journal of Happiness Studies: An Interdisciplinary Forum on Subjective Well-Being*, 6(1), 25–41.

the more fulfillment ... Rogatko, T.P. (2009). "The influence of flow on positive affect in college students." *Journal of Happiness Studies: An Interdisciplinary Forum on Subjective Well-Being*, 10(2), 133–148.

Chapter 1

167,000 fans ... "Track Town Olympic Trials Attendance Hits the Mark," TracktownUSA.com.

Sometimes you hit this flow ... Goucher, K. Author interview 22 March 2019.

But after more than a decade ... Goucher, K. (2017) "How a trip to run a race back home reinvigorated my love for running," https://www.motivrunning.com/running-life/the-voice-of-the-athlete/kara-goucher-finding-way-back-home/> [Accessed January 2019]

Instead of driving ... Permission to use granted by Kara Goucher, https://www.motivrunning.com/running-life/the-voice-of-the-athlete/kara-goucher-finding-way-back-home/> [Accessed January 2019]

The emergence of research ... Csikszentmihalyi, M. (2008), *Flow: The Psychology of Optimal Experience*, New York: Harper Perennial Modern Classics.

Others prefer less religious ... Laski, M. (1990), *Ecstasy in Secular and Religious Experience*, Los Angeles: J.P. Tarcher.

environmental psychologist ... Chawla, L. (1990). "Ecstatic places." *Children's Environments Quarterly*, 7(4), 18–23.

In their 1978 book ... Murphy, M. and White, R.A. (1995), *In the Zone: Transcendent Experience in Sports*, London: Penguin Books.

descriptions of optimal experience ... Maslow, A.H. (1994). *Religions, Values, and Peak Experiences*, London: Penguin Books.

famous French explorer ... David-Neel, A. (1971), *Magic and Mystery in Tibet*, New York: Dover.

In his study of runners ... Glasser, W. (1985), *Positive Addiction*, New York: Harper Colophon Books.

state of exaltation … Laski, M. (1990), *Ecstasy in Secular and Religious Experience*, Los Angeles: J.P. Tarcher.

running-induced euphoria … Lilliefors, J. (1978). *The Running Mind*, Mountain View, CA: World Publications.

After spending two years … Ronkainen, N. and Ryba, T.V. "That is why I gave in to age my competitive ability, but not my soul! A Spiritual Journey in Endurance Running." *Journal for the Study of Spirituality*, 2:1, 10–28, (2012). Granted permission to use February 2019.

third wind … Macauley, I.T. "Marathon Men and Women on Their Marks," New York Times, 22 October 1976.

The first sub-four … Bannister, R. (2004), *The Four-Minute Mile*, New York: Lyons Press.

When I surveyed … Author survey conducted December 2018.

I would describe … Wardian, M. Author interview 2 February 2019.

a full 77 percent … Sachs, M.H. (1980). "On the trail of the runner's high: A descriptive and experimental investigation of characteristics of an elusive phenomenon." Doctoral dissertation, Florida State University.

drug-induced highs … Mandell, A.J. (1981). "The second wind." In M.H. Sacks and M.L. Sachs (Eds.), *Psychology of Running* (pp. 221–223). Champaign, IL: Human Kinetics

at least 27 different … Sachs, M.H. (1980). "On the trail of the runner's high: A descriptive and experimental investigation of characteristics of an elusive phenomenon." Doctoral dissertation, Florida State University.

feelings of exaltation … Sharat G. and Shallu, M. (2015). "Runner's high: A review of the plausible mechanisms underlying exercise-induced ecstasy." *Saudi Journal of Sports Medicine*, 15:3, 207–209.

joy, relaxation and … Fuss J. et al. (2015). "A runner's high depends on cannabinoid receptors in mice." Proceedings of the National Academy of Sciences of the United States of America.

In the flow state … Sherlin, L. Author interview 8 January 2019.

major role in motivating … Stoll, O. (2018). "Peak Performance, the Runner's High, and Flow." in *Handbook of Sports and Exercise Psychology*, American Psychology Association.

major role in motivating … Raichlen, D.A. et al. (2012). "Wired to run: exercise-induced endocannabinoid signaling in humans and cursorial mammals with implication for the runner's high." *Journal of Experimental Biology*, 215: 1331–1336.

What runners say … Author survey conducted December 2018.

electrical, chemical, and architectural … As discussed with Leslie Sherlin, December 2018.

We theorize that … Sherlin, L. Author interview 8 January 2019.

border of alpha and theta … Dietrich, A. (2004). "Neurocognitive mechanisms underlying the experience of flow." *Consciousness and Cognition*, 13(4): 746–61.

neurochemicals might be involved … Hinton E.R. and Taylor, S. "Does placebo response mediate runner's high." *Perceptual and Motor Skills*, 62(3): 789–90.

chase down predators … Raichlen D.A. et al. (2012). "Wired to run: exercise-induced endocannabinoid signaling in humans and cursorial mammals with implication for the runner's high." *Journal of Experimental Biology*, 215: 1331–1336.

Even back in the 1980s … Glasser, W. (1985), *Positive Addiction*, New York: Harper Colophon Books.

Transient hypofrontality … Dietrich, A. (2003). "Functional neuroanatomy of altered states of consciousness: The transient hypofrontality hypothesis." *Consciousness and Cognition*, 12 (2):231–256.

specific elements that characterize … Csikszentmihalyi, M. (2008), *Flow: The Psychology of Optimal Experience*, New York: Harper Perennial Modern Classics. He identifies nine elements of flow.

need be present … Sugiyama T. and Inomata K. (2005). "Qualitative examination of flow experience among top Japanese athletes." *Perceptual Motor Skills*, 100: 969–82.

I've found that … Conley, K. Author interview 16 February 2017, quoted in M.L. Havey, *Mindful Running* (2017).

When I'm running … Pappas, A. Author interview 23 March 2017, quoted in M.L. Havey, *Mindful Running* (2017).

When I am in the zone … Ahmed, M. Author interview 1 March 2017, quoted in M.L. Havey, *Mindful Running* (2017).

It's a quasi … Pollock, P. Author interview 22 March 2017, quoted in M.L. Havey, *Mindful Running* (2017).

I think in … Petty, A. Author interview 14 March 2017, quoted in M.L. Havey, *Mindful Running* (2017).

If you practice … Kastor, D. Author interview 4 April 2017, quoted in M.L. Havey, *Mindful Running* (2017).

calculated amount of stress … Dhabhar, F.S. (2014). "Effects of stress on immune function: the good, the bad, and the beautiful." *Journal of Immunology Research*, 58 (2–3): 193–210.

overly competitive environment … Glasser, W. (1985), *Positive Addiction*, New York: Harper Colophon Books.

self-judgment and endless evaluation … Kostrubala, T. (2013), *The Joy of Running*, St. Nicholas Productions.

Chapter 2

Markus Torgeby … Torgeby, M. (2018), *The Runner: Four Years Living and Running in the Wilderness*, London: Bloomsbury Sport.

spinning around in … Schwartz, C. "How to Hack Your Brain," *The New York Times*, 21 September 2017.

anthropologist Allen Abramson … Lockwood, A. "Running and academia: The intellectual aspect of pounding the pavements," *The Guardian*, 30 June 2014.

legendary track star … Jordan, T. (1997), *Pre: The Story of America's Greatest Running Legend, Steve Prefontaine*, Pennsylvania: Rodale Books.

When we run … Shainberg, D. (1977). "Long distance running as meditation." *Annals of the New York Academy of Sciences*, 301: 1002–1009.

hard fun … Papert, S. "How to make writing 'hard fun,'" *Bangor Daily News*, 24 June 2002.

perceived challenge is a strong ... Abuhamdeh, S. and Csikszentmihalyi, M. (2012). "The importance of challenge for the enjoyment of intrinsically motivated, goal-directed activities." *Personality and Social Psychology Bulletin*, 38(3):317–30.

runners of all paces ... Thum, J.S. et al. (2017). "High-intensity interval training elicits higher enjoyment than moderate intensity continuous exercise," *PLOS One.*

motivated to repeatedly complete ... Csikszentmihalyi, M. and LeFevre, J. (1989). "Optimal Experience in Work and Leisure." *Journal of Personality and Social Psychology*, 56(5):815–822.

calculated amount of stress ... Dhabhar, F.S. (2014). "Effects of stress on immune function: the good, the bad, and the beautiful." *Journal of Immunology Research*, 58 (2–3): 193–210.

overly competitive environment ... Glasser, W. (1985), *Positive Addiction*, New York: Harper Colophon Books.

George Sheehan argued ... Sheehan, G. (2014), *Running & Being: The Total Experience*, Pennsylvania: Rodale Books.

In her memoir ... Kastor, D. (2018), *Let Your Mind Run: A Memoir of Thinking My Way to Victory*, New York: Crown Archetype.

scholarly study of play ... Huizinga, J. (2016), *Homo Ludens: A Study of the Play-Element in Culture*, New York: Angelico Press.

I start to run ... Torgeby, M. (2018), *The Runner: Four Years Living and Running in the Wilderness*, London: Bloomsbury Sport.

One of my favorite ... Lobby, M. "Smash Face Runners and Hooligans," *Marathon and Beyond*, June 2011.

experts suggest that ... Csikszentmihalyi, M. (2000), *Beyond Boredom and Anxiety*, New York: Jossey-Bass.

Chapter 3

I caught up with her ... Lobby, Mackenzie. "Zoe Romano reinvents Tour de France," espnW, 3 July 2014.

concept largely introduced ... Kabat-Zinn, J. (2013), *Full Catastrophe Living*, New York: Bantam.

Renowned Danish thinker ... Kierkegaard, S. (1992), *Either/Or: A Fragment of Life*, New York: Penguin Classics.

spend more than half ... Killingsworth, M.A. and Gilbert, D.T. (2010), "A wandering mind is an unhappy mind." *Science*, 330 (6006): 932.

tend to be happiest ... Killingsworth, M.A. and Gilbert, D.T. (2010), "A wandering mind is an unhappy mind." *Science*, 330 (6006): 932.

Mindfulness gives you a flashlight ... Taren, A. Author interview 15 March 2017, quoted in M.L. Havey, *Mindful Running* (2017).

It can be hard ... Sherlin, L. Author interview 8 January 2019.

Being open to the ... Romano, Z. Author interview 15 February 2019.

as little as six ... Aherne, C., Moran, A. P., and Lonsdale, C. (2011). "The effect of mindfulness training on athletes' flow: An initial investigation." *The Sport Psychologist*, 25(2): 177–189.

likelihood an athlete ... Kee, Y. H. and Wang, C.K.J. (2008). "Relationships between mindfulness, flow dispositions and mental skills adoption: A cluster analytic approach." *Psychology of Sport and Exercise*, 9(4): 393–411.

review of the current … Swann, C. et al. (2012). "A systemic review of the experience, occurrence, and controllability of flow states in elite sport." *Psychology of Sport and Exercise*, 13(6): 807–819.

just five days … Menezes, C.B. and Bizarro, L. (2015). "Effects of focused meditation on difficulties in emotion regulation and trait anxiety." *Psychology & Neuroscience*, 8(3): 350–365.

conscientiousness rose to … Ullen, F. and Almeida, R. (2012). "Proneness for psychological flow in everyday life: Associations with personality and intelligence." *Personality and Individual Differences*, 52(2).

I've found flow … Joyner, M. Author interview 1 February 2019.

Emotional intelligence has … Srinivasan, N. and Gingras, B. (2014). "Emotional intelligence predicts individual differences in proneness for flow among musicians: the role of control and distributed attention." *Frontiers in Psychology*, 4:853.

Three main ways … Charoensukmongkol, P. (2014). "Benefits of mindfulness meditation on emotional intelligence, general self-efficacy, and perceived stress: Evidence from Thailand." *Journal of Spirituality in Mental Health*, 16(3): 171–192.

one study on emotional … Rubaltelli, E. et al. (2018). "Emotional intelligence impact on half marathon finish times." *Personality and Individual Differences*, 128: 107–112.

affect labeling … Lieberman, M.D. et al. (2007). "Putting feelings into words: affect labeling disrupts amygdala activity in response to affective stimuli." *Psychological Science*, 18(5): 421–428.

mindfulness can increase … Ruffault, A. et al. (2016). "Mindfulness may moderate the relationship between intrinsic motivation and physical activity: A cross-sectional study." *Mindfulness*, 7(2): 445–452.

Mindfulness helps athletes … Mahmood, D. et al. (2018). "Effectiveness of the mindfulness-acceptance-commitment-based approach on athletic performance and sports competition anxiety: A randomized clinical trial." *Electronic Physician*, 10(5): 6749–6755.

NCAA athletes … Goodman, F.R. et al. (2014). "A brief mindfulness and yoga intervention with an entire NCAA Division I athletic team: An initial investigation." *Psychology of Consciousness: Theory, Research, and Practice*, 1(4): 339–356.

open and receptive attitude … Carpenter, J.K. et al. (2018). "The effect of a brief mindfulness training on distress tolerance and stress reactivity." *Behavior Therapy*, 50(3): 630–645.

Mindfully cultivated … Basu, A. et al. (2018). "Attention Restoration Theory: Exploring the role of soft fascination and mental bandwidth." *Environment and Behavior*, 51(9–10).

feeling of awe … Keltner, D. and Haidt, J. (2010). "Approaching awe, a moral, spiritual, and aesthetic emotion." *Cognition and Emotion*, 17(2): 297–314.

feeling of connection … Stellar, J.E. (2015). "Positive affect and markers of inflammation: Discrete positive emotions predict lower levels of inflammatory cytokines." *Emotion*, 15(2): 129–133.

increase happiness… Kini, P. et al. (2016). "The effects of gratitude expression on neural activity." *NeuroImage*, 128(1): 1-10.

and optimism ... Emmons, R.A. and McCullough, M.E. (2003). "Counting blessings versus burdens: An experimental investigation of gratitude and subjective well-being in daily life." *Journal of Personality and Social Psychology*, 84(2): 377–389.

naturally deactivate a ... Zeidan, F. (2018). "Neural mechanisms supporting the relationship between dispositional mindfulness and pain." *Pain*, 159(12): 2477–2485.

focused on process ... Jackson, S.A. and Roberts, G.C. (1992). "Positive performance states of athletes: Toward a conceptual understanding of peak performance." *The Sport Psychologist*, 6(2): 156–171.

Arne Dietrich ... Dietrich, A. and Stoll, O. (2010). "Effortless attention, hypofrontality, and perfectionism." In B. Bruya (Ed.), *Effortless attention: A new perspective in the cognitive science of attention and action* (pp. 159–178). Cambridge, MA, US: MIT Press.

Mindset: The New ... Dweck, C. (2007), *Mindset: The New Psychology of Success*, New York: Ballantine Books.

overly concerned about ... Jackson, S.A. and Roberts, G.C. (1992). "Positive performance states of athletes: Toward a conceptual understanding of peak performance." *The Sport Psychologist*, 6(2): 156–171.

people open to new ... Phares, E.J. and Chaplin, W.F. (1997), *Introduction to Personality*, 4th Edition.

flow-inducing tasks ... De Fruyt, F., De Wiele, L.V., and Van Heeringen, C. (2000). "Cloninger's psychobiological model of temperament and character and the Five-Factor Model of personality." *Personality and Individual Differences*, 29(3), 441–452.

Openness is also ... Steel, P. et al. (2008). "Refining the relationship between personality and subjective well-being." *Psychology Bulletin*, 134(1): 138–161.

my first book ... Havey, M.L. (2017), *Mindful Running*, London: Bloomsbury Sport.

neurons that fire ... Hebb, D.O. (1949), *The Organization of Behavior*, New York: Wiley.

Achieving flow ... Keflezighi, M. Author interview 14 March 2017, quoted in M.L. Havey, *Mindful Running* (2017).

systematic reviews of ... Swann, C. et al. (2012). "A systematic review of the experience, occurrence, and controllability of flow states in elite sport." *Psychology of Sport and Exercise*, 13(6): 807–819.

We want to ... Gervais, M. Author interview 9 August 2017.

With greater awareness ... Gervais, M. Author interview 9 August 2017.

Laurence Gonzales ... Gonzales, L. (2004), *Deep Survival: Who Lives, Who Dies, and Why*, New York: W.W. Norton & Company.

Chapter 4

No matter what ... Van Deren, D. Author interview 21 March 2019.

The Atlantic ... Havey, M. "Running From the Seizures," *The Atlantic*, 12 December 2014.

intrinsic motivation as ... Maslow, A. (1994), *Religions, Values, and Peak-Experiences*, New York: Penguin Books.

harmonious passion … Vallerand, R.J. et al. (2003). "On obsessive and harmonious passion." *Journal of Personality and Social Psychology*, 85(4): 756–767.

first-time marathoners … Schuler, J. and Brunner, S. (2009). "The rewarding effect of flow experience on performance in a marathon race." *Psychology of Sport and Exercise*, 10: 168–174.

persistence is key … Baumann, N. and Scheffer, D. (2011). "Seeking flow in the achievement domain: The achievement flow motive behind flow experience." *Motivation and Emotion*, 35: 267–284.

Self-Determination Theory … Ryan, R.M. and Deci, E.L. (2000). "Self-determination theory and the facilitation of intrinsic motivation, social development, and well-being." *American Psychologist*, 55(1): 68–78.

meeting these needs … Kowal J. and Fortier, M.S. (1999) "Motivational determinants of flow: Contributions from self-determination theory." *The Journal of Social Psychology*, 139(3): 355–368.

Once these basic … Deci, E.L., (1992). "The relation of interest to the motivation of behavior: A self-determination theory perspective" in Renninger, K.A., Hidi, S., Krapp, A. (Eds.). *The Role of Interest in Learning and Development* (pp. 43–70). Hillsdale, NJ, US: Lawrence Erlbaum Associates, Inc.

interest plays a … O'Keefe, P.A. et al. (2017). "The multifaceted role of interest in motivation and engagement" in O'Keefe, P.A. and Harackiewicz, J.M. (Eds.). *The Science of Interest*.

interest plays a … Thoman, D.B. et al. (2017). "The dynamic nature of interest: Embedding interest within self-regulation" in O'Keefe, P.A. and Harackiewicz, J.M. (Eds.). *The Science of Interest*.

Famed American philosopher … Dewey, J. (1913), *Interest and Effort in Education*, Boston: Houghton Mifflin Co.

Research backs up the fact… O'Keefe, P.A. and Linnenbrink-Garcia, L. (2014). "The role of interest in optimizing performance and self-regulation." *Journal of Experimental Social Psychology*, 53: 70–78.

long-term study … Ogas, O. "The Dark Horse Project," Harvard University.

True North Goals … Havey, M.L. (2017), *Mindful Running*, London: Bloomsbury Sport.

taking time not only to … Chase, J.A. et al. (2013). "Values are not just goals: Online ACT-based values training adds to goal setting in improving undergraduate college student performance." *Journal of Contextual Behavioral Science*, 2: 79–84.

In interviews since … Miller, N. "Q&A With Joan Benoit Samuelson, 30 Years After Gold," *Podium Runner*, 2014.

imagery exercises … Morris, T. et al. 2005, *Imagery in Sport*, Champaign, IL: Human Kinetics.

visualization can impact … Koehn, S. and Díaz-Ocejo, J. (2016). "Imagery intervention to increase flow state: A single-case study with middle-distance runners in the state of Qatar." *International Journal of Sport and Exercise Psychology*, 1–14.

open to fresh … Langer, E.J. (2000). "Mindful Learning." *Current Directions in Psychological Science*, 9(6).

interpreting experiences … Wilson, T.D. (2015), *Redirect: Changing the Stories We Live By*, Boston: Back Bay Books.

inner narrative and … Turnwald, B.P. (2018). "Learning one's genetic risk changes physiology independent of actual genetic risk." *Nature Human Behaviour*, 3: 48–56.

What runners say … Author survey conducted December 2018.

A keen awareness … Brown, K.W. and Ryan, R.M. (2003). "The benefits of being present: Mindfulness and its role in psychological well-being." *Journal of Personality and Social Psychology*, 84(4): 822–848.

greater authenticity … Leroy, H. et al. (2013). "Mindfulness, authentic functioning, and work engagement: A growth modeling approach." *Journal of Vocational Behavior*, 82(3): 238–247.

embodied cognition … Cuddy, A.J. et al. (2018). "P-curving a more comprehensive body of research on postural feedback reveals clear evidential value for power-posing effects: Reply to Simmons and Simonsohn." *Psychological Science*, 29(4).

In the 1970s … Bandura, A. (1994). Self-efficacy. In V.S. Ramachaudran (Ed.), Encyclopedia of human behavior (Vol. 4, pp. 71–81). New York: Academic Press. (Reprinted in H. Friedman [Ed.], *Encyclopedia of Mental Health*. San Diego: Academic Press, 1998).

Not only do … McCormick, A. et al. (2017). "Effects of a motivational self-talk intervention for endurance athletes completing an ultramarathon." *The Sport Psychologist*, 32(1): 42–50.

While we all … Breines, J.G. and Chen, S. (2012). "Self-compassion increases self-improvement motivation." *Personality and Social Psychology Bulletin*, 38(9).

self-compassion has … Ferguson, L.J. et al. (2014). "Exploring self-compassion and eudaimonic well-being in young women athletes." *Journal of Sport & Exercise Psychology*, 36: 203–216.

self-compassion and exercise motivation … Magnus, C.M. and Kowalski, K.C. (2010). "The role of self-compassion in women's self-determined motives to exercise and exercise-related outcomes." *Self and Identity*, 9: 363–382.

Socratic questioning … Seppala, E. (2016), *The Happiness Track*, New York: HarperOne.

Chapter 5

Just moments before … Keflezighi, M. and Douglas, S. (2019), *26 Marathons: What I Learned About Faith, Identity, Running, and Life from My Marathon Career*, Pennsylvania: Rodale Books.

Born in Eritrea … Keflezighi, M. (2014), *Run to Overcome: The Inspiring Story of an American Champion's Long-Distance Quest to Achieve a Big Dream*, Chicago: Tyndale Momentum.

I can't even … Keflezighi, M. Author interview 14 May 2017, quoted in M.L. Havey, *Mindful Running* (2017).

A report published … Ordóñez, L.D. et al. (2009). "Goals Gone Wild: The systematic side effects of over-prescribing goal setting." *Harvard Business School Review*.

People report being … Csikszentmihalyi, M. (2008), *Flow: The Psychology of Optimal Experiences*, New York: Harper Perennial.

According to some ... Heinrich, B. (2002), *Why We Run*, New York: Harper Perennial.

when mice adeptly ... Goto, Y. and Grace A.A. (2005). "Dopaminergic modulation of limbic and cortical drive of nucleus accumbens in goal-directed behavior." *Nature Neuroscience*, 8(6): 805–812.

when mice adeptly ... Howe, M.W. et al. (2013). "Prolonged Dopamine Signalling in Striatum Signals Proximity and Value of Distant Rewards." *Nature*, 500(7464): 575–579.

a researcher of human ... Fogg, B.J. bjfogg.com.

S.M.A.R.T. Goals ... Doran, G.T. (1981). "There's a S.M.A.R.T. way to write management's goals and objectives." *Management Review*, 70(11): 35–36.

remember to jot ... Weinberg, R. (2010). "Making Goals Effective: A Primer for Coaches." *Journal of Sport Psychology in Action*, 1(2): 57–65.

physiology is affected ... Kiely, J. (2016). "Essay: A new understanding of stress and the implications for our cultural training paradigm." *New Studies in Athletics*, 34: 69–74.

What runners say ... Author survey conducted December 2018.

proper hydration could ... Davis, B.A. et al. (2014). "Hydration kinetics and 10-km outdoor running performance following 75% versus 150% between bout fluid replacement." *European Journal of Sports Science*, 14(7): 703–710.

a small decrement ... Casa, D.J. et al. (2010). "Influence of hydration on physiological function and performance during trail running in the heat." *Journal of Athletic Training*, 45(2): 147–156.

solid eight hours ... "Extra Sleep Could Improve Athletic Performance." National Sleep Foundation.

illuminated by new ... Kiely, J. (2016). "Essay: A new understanding of stress and the implications for our cultural training paradigm." *New Studies in Athletics*, 34: 69–74.

Chapter 6

In a 2008 essay ... Burfoot, A. "Running Scared," *Runner's World*, 5 May 2008.

In a 2004 ... Burfoot, A. "Runner's High," *Runner's World*, 28 April 2004.

Training was smooth ... Burfoot, A. "Running Scared," *Runner's World*, 5 May 2008.

He took stock ... Burfoot, A. "Running Scared," *Runner's World*, 5 May 2008.

I surged just ... Burfoot, A. Author interview, 18 March 2019.

The early literature ... Glasser, W. (1985), *Positive Addiction*, New York: Harper Colophon Books.

What runners say ... Author survey conducted December 2018.

decision fatigue ... Brocas, I. and Carrillo, J.D. (Eds.) (2002), *The Psychology of Economic Decisions*, Oxford: Oxford University Press.

believe that willpower ... Muraven, M. (2010). "Building self-control strength: Practicing self-control leads to improved self-control performance." *Journal of Experimental Social Psychology*, 46(2): 465–468.

the most convincing ... Lally, P. et al. (2010). "How are habits formed: Modelling habit formation in the real world." *European Journal of Social Psychology*, 40(6): 998–1009.

scenario planning ... Chermack, T.J. (2005). "Studying scenario planning: Theory, research suggestions, and hypotheses." *Technological Forecasting and Social Change*, 72(1): 59–73.

seeing yourself from ... Patrick, V.M. et al. (2009). "Affective forecasting and self-control: Why anticipating pride wins over anticipating shame in a self-regulation context." *Journal of Consumer Psychology*, 19(3): 537–545.

exercise is a foundational ... Blair, S.N. et al. (1985). "Relationships between exercise or physical activity and other health behaviors." *Public Health Reports*, 100(2): 172–180.

competitive athletes identify ... Russell, W.D. (2001). "An examination of flow state occurrence in college athletes." *Journal of Sport Behavior*, 24: 83.

Dr. Cindra Kamphoff ... Kamphoff, C. (2017), *Beyond Grit: Ten Powerful Practices to Gain the High-Performance Edge*, Minneapolis, Wise Ink Creative Publishing.

Total absorption in ... Lobby, M. "Getting in the (pre-race) zone," *Triathlete*, 17 August 2015.

finding that purposely ... Massi, B. et al. (2018). "Volatility facilitates value updating in the prefrontal cortex." *Neuron*, 99(3): 598–608.

A pioneer when ... Bridel, W. et al. (Eds.) (2015), *Endurance Running: A Socio-Cultural Examination*, Abingdon: Routledge.

early forms of ... Bale, J. (2003), *Running Cultures*, Abingdon: Routledge.

deliberate practice ... Ericsson, A. and Pool, R. (2016), *Peak: Secrets from the New Science of Expertise*, New York: Houghton Mifflin Harcourt.

anywhere from 40 ... Carrell, S.E. et al. (2010). "Is poor fitness contagious? Evidence from randomly assigned friends." The National Bureau of Economic Research, No. 16518.

rate of perceived exertion ... Van Erp, T. et al. (2019). "Relationship between various training-load measures in elite cyclists during training, road races, and time trials." *International Journal of Sports Physiology and Performance*, 14(4): 493–500.

Leveraging the power ... Haase, L. et al. (2015). "A pilot study investigating changes in neural processing after mindfulness training in elite athletes." *Frontiers in Behavioral Neuroscience*, 9: 229.

Mindfulness can help ... Hecht, R. Author interview 15 March 2017, quoted in M.L. Havey, *Mindful Running* (2017).

Your rate of ... "Rated Perceived Exertion (RPE) Scale," Cleveland Clinic.

Here's a quick ... Borg, G.A. (1982). "Psychophysical bases of perceived exertion." *Medicine & Science in Sports & Exercise*, 14(5): 377–381.

Chapter 7

In late January ... "One Team, One Goal," https://www.nazelite.com/video/one-team-one-goal-episode-3-the-workout/>

When we arrived ... Taylor, K. Author interview 26 February 2019.

We didn't really ... Smith, S. Author interview 26 February 2019.

I vividly remember ... Rosario, B. Author interview 8 February 2019.

landmark story ... Sillitoe, A. (1959), *The Loneliness of the Long-Distance Runner*, New York: Vintage Books.

If you're having ... McMillan, G.. Author interview 4 February 2019.

social flow experiences ... Walker, C. (2010). "Experiencing flow: Is doing it together better than doing it alone?" *The Journal of Positive Psychology*, 5(1): 3–11.

cultural anthropology ... Olaveson, T. (2001). "Collective effervescence and communitas: Processual models of ritual and society in Emile Durkheim and Victor Turner." *Dialectical Anthropology*, 26: 105.

As it turns ... Jackson, S.A. and Csikszentmihalyi, M. (1999), *Flow in sports: The keys to optimal experiences and performances*, Champaign, IL: Human Kinetics Books.

Social Facilitation suggests ... Strube, M.J. et al. (1981). "The social facilitation of a simple task: Field tests of alternative explanations." *Personality and Social Psychology Bulletin*, 7(4): 701–707.

Emotional Contagion Theory ... Bavelas, J.B. et al. (1987). "Motor mimicry as primitive empathy" In Eisenberg N. and Strayer J. (Eds.), *Cambridge Studies in Social and Emotional Development: Empathy and its Development*, 317–338. New York: Cambridge University Press.

agents of flow ... Salanova, M. et al. (2014). "Flowing together: A longitudinal study of collective efficacy and collective flow among workgroups." *The Journal of Psychology*, 148(4): 435–455.

Many of the factors ... Pels, F. et al. (2018). "Group flow: A scoping review of definitions, theoretical approaches, measures and findings." *PLOS One*.

Many of the factors ... Sawyer, K. (2008), *Group Genius: The Creative Power of Collaboration*, New York: Basic Books.

process of discussing ... O'Leary-Kelly, A.M. et al. (1994). "A review of the influence of group goals on group performance." *The Academy of Management Journal*, 37(5): 1285–1301.

individual runners focus ... Weick, K.E. and Roberts, K. H. (1993). "Collective mind in organizations: Heedful interrelating on flight decks." *Administrative Science Quarterly*, 38(3): 357–381.

the following three ... Martin, E.M. et al. (2017). "Developing a team mission statement: Who are we? Where are we going? How are we going to get there?" *Journal of Sport Psychology in Action*, 8(3): 197–207.

Experts suggest that ... Cosma, J.B. (1999), "Flow in Teams." Doctoral dissertation, *Chicago School of Professional Psychology*.

when you believe ... Humphrey, S.E. et al. (2007). "Integrating motivational, social, and contextual work design features: A meta-analytic summary and theoretical extension of the work design literature." *Journal of Applied Psychology*, 92(5): 1332–1356.

team cohesion is ... Lazarovitz, S. M. (2003). "Team and individual flow in female ice hockey players: The relationships between flow, group cohesion, and athletic performance." University of Calgary, Thesis.

Social Identity Theory ... Ashforth, B.E. and Mael, F. (1989). "Social identity theory and the organization." *Academy of Management Review*, 14(1): 20–39.

Social Identity Theory ... Tajfel, H. (2010), *Social Identity and Intergroup Relations*, Cambridge University Press.

social psychology literature ... Carron, A.V. and Spink, K.S. (1995). "The group size-cohesion relationship in minimal groups." *Small Group Research*, 26(1).

Identity may arise ... Zaccaro, S.J. and McCoy, M.C. (1988). "The effects of task and interpersonal cohesiveness on performance of a disjunctive group task." *Journal of Applied Social Psychology*, 18(10): 837–851.

Collective efficacy … Salanova, M. et al. (2014). "Flowing together: A longitudinal study of collective efficacy and collective flow among workgroups." *The Journal of Psychology*, 148(4): 435–455.

Collective efficacy … Ballesteros-Fernández, R. et al. (2002). "Determinants and structural relation of personal efficacy to collective efficacy." *Applied Psychology: An International Review*, 51(1): 107–125.

there needs to … Salanova, M. et al. (2014). "Flowing together: A longitudinal study of collective efficacy and collective flow among workgroups." *The Journal of Psychology*, 148(4): 435–455.

Spanish researchers confirmed … Salanova, M. et al. (2014). "Flowing together: A longitudinal study of collective efficacy and collective flow among workgroups." *The Journal of Psychology*, 148(4): 435–455.

This is probably … Van Den Hout, J.J. et al. (2017). "The conceptualization of team flow." *The Journal of Psychology*, 152(6): 388–423.

Individual self-efficacy … Sánchez, A. et al. (2011). "When good is good: A virtuous circle of self-efficacy and flow at work among teachers." *Revista de Psicología Social*, 26.

Positive Group Affect Spiral … Walter, F. and Bruch, H. (2008). "The positive group affect spiral: A dynamic model of the emergence of positive affective similarity in work groups." *Journal of Organizational Behavior*, 29(2): 239–261.

A motivational environment … Aube, C. et al. (2013). "Flow experience and team performance: The role of team goal commitment and information exchange." *Motivation and Emotion*, 38(1): 120–130.

Intrinsic motivation is … Walker, C. (2010). "Experiencing flow: Is doing it together better than doing it alone?" *The Journal of Positive Psychology*, 5(1): 3–11.

Shared intrinsic motivation … Ready, D.A. and Truelove, E. (2011). "The power of collective ambition." *Harvard Business Review*, 89(12): 94–102.

believe that collective … Hackman, J.R. and Wageman, R. (2005). "A theory of team coaching." *Academy of Management Review*, 30(2).

it can augment … Stewart, G. (2006). "A meta-analytic review of relationships between team design features and team performance." *Journal of Management*, 32(1).

Collective flow experiences … Bandura, A. (1982). "Self-efficacy mechanism in human agency." *American Psychologist*, 37(2): 122–147.

When team members … Lencioni, P. (2002), *The Five Dysfunctions of a Team: A Leadership Fable*, San Francisco: Jossey-Bass.

This encourages greater … Bakker, A.B. et al. (2011). "Flow and performance: A study among talented Dutch soccer players." *Psychology of Sport and Exercise*, 12(4): 442–450.

The synergistic nature … Van Den Hout, J.J. et al. (2017). "The conceptualization of team flow." *The Journal of Psychology*, 152(6): 388–423.

Chapter 8

World Marathon Challenge … www.worldmarathonchallenge.com>

I just accepted… Wardian, M. Author interview 2 February 2019.

Studies from the 1980s … Wagemaker, H. and Goldstein, L. (1980). "The runner's high." *The Journal of Sports Medicine and Physical Fitness*, 20. 227–9.

kind of high priest … Van Doorn, J. "An Intimidating New Class: The Physical Elite," *New York Magazine*, 29 May 1978.

ultramarathoners measured … Wollseiffen, P. et al. (2016). "The effect of 6 h of running on brain activity, mood, and cognitive performance." *Experimental Brain Research*, 234(7): 1829–1836.

some level of running … Stoll, O. (2018). "Peak performance, the runner's high and flow" in *Handbook of Sports and Exercise Psychology*, American Psychology Association.

perfection is in … Hicks, S.D. et al. (2019). "The transcriptional signature of a runner's high." *Medicine & Science in Sports & Exercise*, 51(5): 970–978.

Pulitzer Prize-winning … Wilson, E.O. (1984), *Biophilia*, Boston: Harvard University Press.

it can reduce … Li, Q. (2018), *Forest Bathing: How Trees Can Help You Find Health and Happiness*, New York: Viking Press.

forest bathing reduces … Park, B.J. et al. (2009). "The physiological effects of Shinrin-yoku (taking in the forest atmosphere or forest bathing): Evidence from field experiments in 24 forests across Japan." *Environmental Health and Preventative Medicine*, 15(1): 18–26.

Researchers in the UK … Aspinall, P. et al. (2015). "The urban brain: Analysing outdoor physical activity with mobile EEG." *British Journal of Sports Medicine*, 49(4): 272–276.

people's brain waves … Raichlen, D.A. (2012). "Wired to run: Exercise-induced endocannabinoid signaling in humans and cursorial mammals with implications for the 'runner's high.'" *Journal of Experimental Biology*, 215(8): 1331–1336.

By 2050 … United Nations, Population Division, https://www.un.org/development/desa/en/news/population/2018-revision-of-world-urbanization-prospects.html>

What runners say … Author survey conducted December 2018.

soft fascination … Kaplan, R. and Kaplan S. (1989), *The Experience of Nature: A Psychological Perspective*, Cambridge: Cambridge University Press.

moving through nature … Aspinall, P. et al. (2015). "The urban brain: Analysing outdoor physical activity with mobile EEG." *British Journal of Sports Medicine*, 49(4): 272–276.

That sense of wonder … Piff, P.K. et al. (2015). "Awe, the small self, and prosocial behavior." *Journal of Personality and Social Psychology*, 108(6): 883–899.

It will come … Csikszentmihalyi, M. (2008), *Flow: The Psychology of Optimal Experience*, New York: Harper Perennial.

Attention Restoration Theory … Kaplan, S. (1995). "The restorative benefits of nature: Toward an integrative framework." *Journal of Environmental Psychology*, 15: 169–182.

discovered that flow … Wöran, B. and Arnberger, A. (2012). "Exploring relationships between recreation specialization, restorative environments and mountain hikers' flow experience." *Leisure Science*, 34(2): 95–114.

natural settings are … Kaplan, R. and Kaplan S. (1989), *The Experience of Nature: A Psychological Perspective*, Cambridge: Cambridge University Press.

conducive to creating … Droit-Volet, S. and Meck, W.H. (2007). "How emotions colour our perception of time." *Trends in Cognitive Science*, 11(12): 504–513.

Chapter 9

By the halfway … Kastor, D. (2018), *Let Your Mind Run: A Memoir of Thinking My Way to Victory*, New York: Crown Archetype.

I was definitely … Kastor, D. Author interview 1 April 2019.

Overtraining syndrome involves … Kreher, J.B. and Schwartz, J.B. (2012). "Overtraining syndrome: A practical guide." *Sports Health*, 4(2): 128–138.

upward of 70 … Hreljac, A. (2004). "Impact and overuse injuries in runners." *Medicine & Science in Sports & Exercise*, 36(5): 845–849.

hard running can … Fitzgerald, L. (1988). "Exercise and the immune system." *Immunology Today*, 9(11): 337–339.

mental fatigue negatively … Van Cutsem, J. et al. (2017). "The effects of mental fatigue on physical performance: A systematic review." *Journal of Sports Medicine*, 47(8): 1569–1588.

seven days following … Hikida, R.S. et al. (1983). "Muscle fiber necrosis associated with human marathon runners." *Journal of the Neurological Sciences*, 59(2): 185–203.

Flow can't be … Kastor, D. Author interview 4 April 2017, quoted in M.L. Havey, *Mindful Running* (2017).

Psychological flexibility … Kashdan, T.B. and Rottenberg, J. (2010). "Psychological flexibility as a fundamental aspect of health." *Clinical Psychology Review*, 30(7): 865–878.

science of neuroplasticity … Begley, S. (2007), *Train Your Mind, Change Your Brain: How a New Science Reveals Our Extraordinary Potential to Transform Ourselves*, New York: Ballantine Books.

poor psychological flexibility … Kato T. (2016). "Impact of psychological inflexibility on depressive symptoms and sleep difficulty in a Japanese sample." *SpringerPlus*, 5(1): 712.

while self-compassion … Magnus, C.M. et al. (2010). "The role of self-compassion in women's self-determined motives to exercise and exercise-related outcomes." *Self and Identity*, 9:363–383.

combat the fear … Mosewich, A.D. et al. (2013). "Applying self-compassion in sport: An intervention with women athletes." *Journal of Sport and Exercise Psychology*, 35: 514–524.

self-compassion may … Breines, J.G. and Chen, S. (2012). "Self-compassion increases self-improvement motivation." *Personality and Social Psychology Bulletin*, 38(9).

Rather than criticizing … Neff, K. D. and Germer, C.K. (2013). "A pilot study and randomized controlled trial of the mindful self-compassion program." *Journal of Clinical Psychology*, 69(1): 28–44.

whereas self-compassion … Kirschner, H. et al. (2019). "Soothing your heart and feeling connected: A new experimental paradigm to study the benefits of self-compassion." *Clinical Psychological Science*, 7(3).

Epilogue

Run a lot … Joyner, M. Granted permission to use 1 February 2019.

INDEX